THE PERIMENOPAUSE PLAN

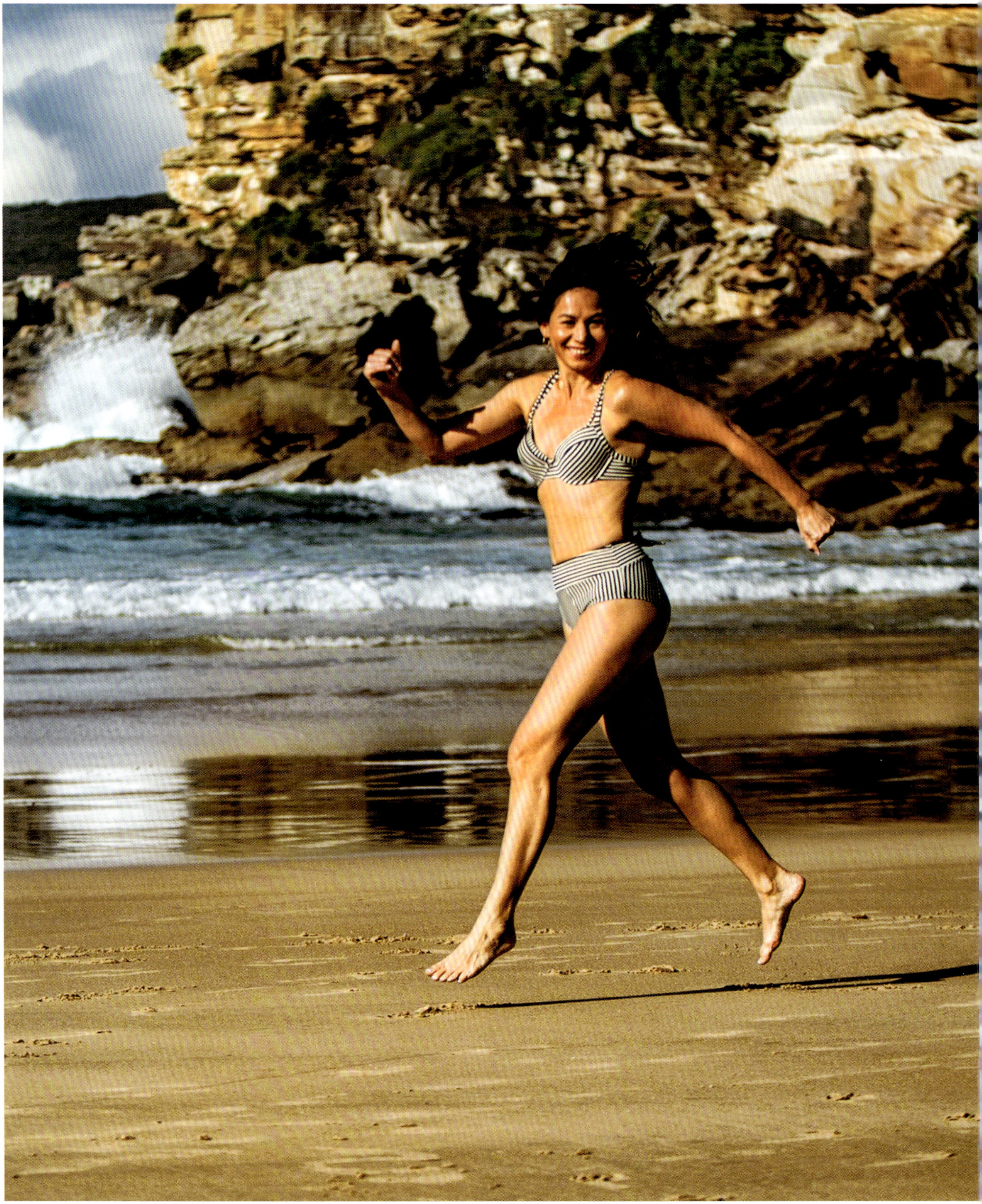

THE PERIMENOPAUSE PLAN

Easy meal plans, 75 recipes, plus key tips to manage weight, regain energy and thrive

FAYE JAMES

NEW HOLLAND

ABOUT THE AUTHOR

FAYE JAMES

Meet Faye James, a leading voice in nutrition, wellness, and women's health. With over two decades of experience, Faye brings a wealth of knowledge and expertise to her work, holding Accreditation as a Nutritionist and memberships with both Nutrition Council Australia and the Australian Menopause Society. Her commitment to empowering women shines through in her extensive writing, speaking engagements, and innovative wellness programs.

Faye is the author of the celebrated *The Long Life Plan* (2018), an anti-ageing recipe book, *The 10:10 Diet* (2019), a popular weight-loss program and recipe eBook, and the bestselling *The Menopause Diet* (2023). Her ability to simplify complex health topics and deliver real, practical solutions has made her a trusted resource for individuals looking to improve their health and well-being.

Faye's expertise has been sought by major brands, including Woolworths, Weight Watchers, Fitness First, and Goodlife. Her writing has appeared in leading publications such as *HELLO! Magazine, ELLE, Body & Soul, Women's Health, Prevention, Glamour,* and *Harper's Bazaar*. Through these platforms, she has inspired countless women to take control of their health journeys.

In her latest book, *The Perimenopause Plan*, Faye turns her focus to a critical yet often overlooked stage of life—perimenopause. Drawing on her extensive research and personal experience managing her own perimenopausal symptoms, Faye provides women with the tools to navigate this transformative phase with confidence. The book combines science-backed advice, practical meal plans, and lifestyle strategies to help women thrive through perimenopause and beyond.

Originally from London, Faye now resides in Sydney with her husband, food photographer Darrin James, and their two children. Passionate about using food as medicine, Faye has dedicated her career to helping women feel their best at every stage of life. Her commitment to health, empowerment, and balance is evident in everything she creates, making *The Perimenopause Plan* an essential resource for women everywhere.

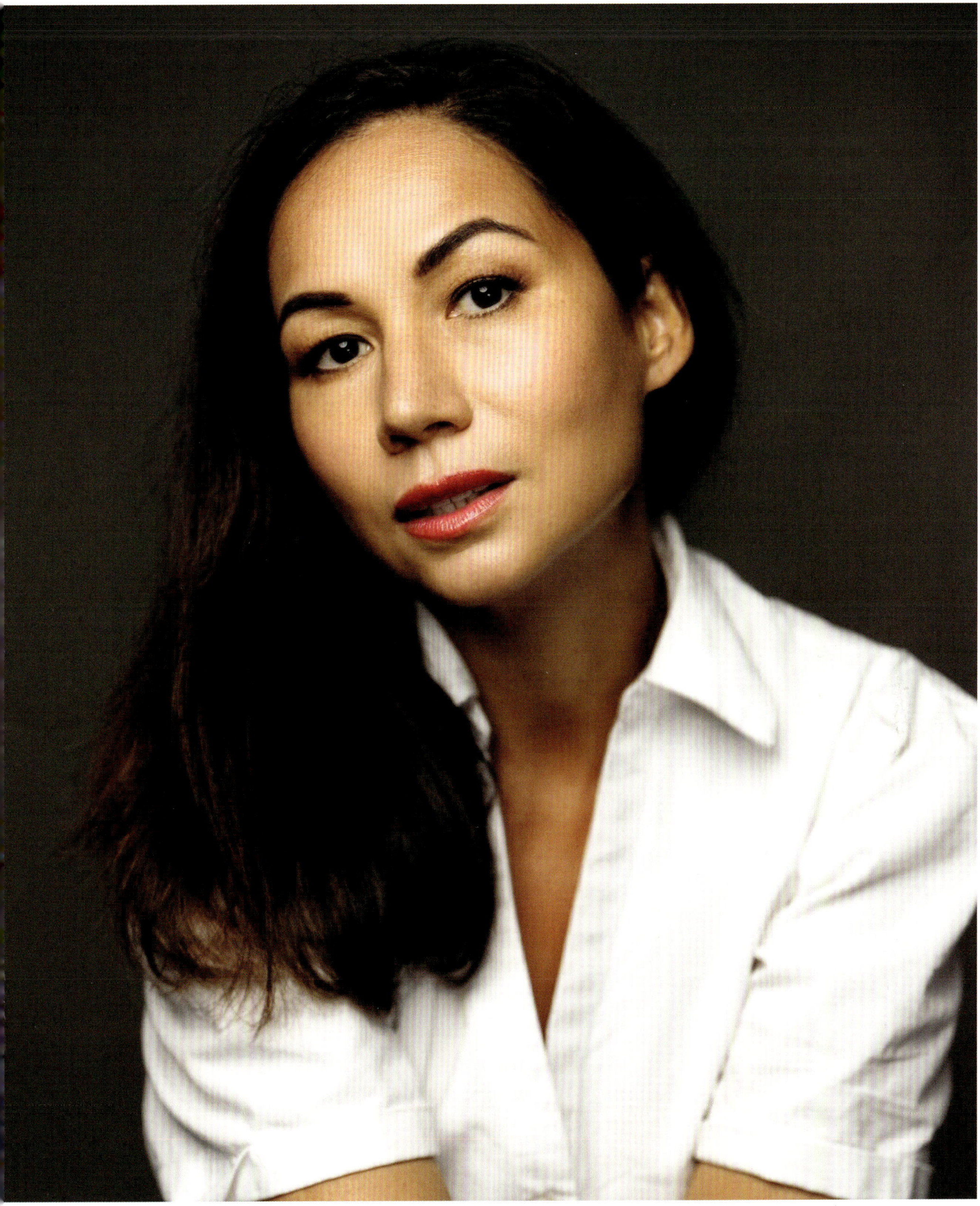

CONTENTS

UNDERSTANDING PERIMENOPAUSE

Perimenopause is the transitional phase leading up to menopause, typically beginning for most women in their late 30s to early 40s. It's a stage characterised by fluctuating hormones – primarily estrogen and progesterone – affecting everything from your energy levels to your mood, sleep, and even your weight. Unlike menopause, which is defined by the absence of menstrual cycles for 12 consecutive months, perimenopause is the precursor where symptoms gradually emerge, often taking women by surprise.

This period may last several years, during which you may experience symptoms like irregular periods, mood swings, weight gain, hot flashes, and sleep disturbances. These changes are a natural part of life, but with the right support, they don't need to derail your lifestyle or sense of well-being.

The power of nutrition and lifestyle

One of the most empowering ways to manage perimenopause is through thoughtful nutrition and lifestyle choices. What we eat, how we move, and the mindfulness practices we adopt can have a profound impact on symptom relief and overall health. Nutrition can help stabilise energy levels, improve mood, aid in weight management, and mitigate symptoms like hot flashes and insomnia. By proactively caring for our bodies through balanced eating, physical activity, and stress management, we can take charge of our health and enjoy this phase with strength.

How can *The Perimenopause Plan* help me?

The Perimenopause Plan is here to guide and support you through this unique time in life. In this book, I've provided comprehensive meal plans, nutritious recipes, and simple lifestyle strategies designed to help you feel empowered, energised, and balanced. Each chapter offers practical tools for a personalised approach to perimenopause. Whether you're looking to boost your energy, stabilise your weight, or improve your mood, this guide has you covered, helping you navigate perimenopause with confidence.

CHAPTER 1

RECOGNISING PERIMENOPAUSE SYMPTOMS AND SETTING GOALS

Understanding your symptoms and setting realistic health goals are the first steps to taking control of perimenopause. For many women, this phase is full of unknowns, and each body reacts differently to hormonal changes. By identifying and tracking your symptoms, you can personalise your approach, setting meaningful goals for your health and wellness during this time.

Identifying common symptoms

Perimenopause often begins subtly, with a few unexpected changes that gradually intensify. The symptoms of perimenopause can vary greatly, but some of the most common include:

- **Irregular periods**: Many women find that their cycles become erratic. Periods may come closer together or further apart, sometimes with heavier or lighter bleeding.
- **Mood swings and irritability**: Hormonal fluctuations can lead to increased anxiety, irritability, or depression, which can feel out of character or overwhelming.
- **Sleep disturbances**: Insomnia, early waking, or interrupted sleep often accompany perimenopause, which in turn affects daily energy levels.
- **Weight gain and changes in body composition**: With shifts in hormone levels, many women notice weight gain, particularly around the abdomen, and find it harder to shed excess weight.
- **Hot flashes and night sweats**: These sudden waves of warmth and perspiration can occur during the day or at night, often disrupting sleep and comfort.
- **Cognitive changes**: Many women experience "brain fog," feeling forgetful or less focused than usual.

Recognising these symptoms and how they uniquely impact you is essential to developing a tailored approach to perimenopause. Knowing your body's reactions allows you to take meaningful steps toward relief and well-being.

Self-assessment

To help you identify and understand your symptoms, I've created a quick self-assessment below. This checklist will give you a clearer picture of your primary concerns and can serve as a reference as you work through this book.

1. How often do you experience mood swings or irritability?

- ○ Frequently
- ○ Occasionally
- ○ Rarely

2. Are you having trouble falling asleep or staying asleep?

- ○ Frequently
- ○ Occasionally
- ○ Rarely

3. Have you noticed unexpected weight gain or changes in body shape, especially around your waist?

- ○ Yes
- ○ No

4. How often do you experience hot flashes or night sweats?

- ○ Frequently
- ○ Occasionally
- ○ Rarely

5. Do you feel more forgetful or unfocused than usual?

- ○ Frequently
- ○ Occasionally
- ○ Rarely

By reviewing these answers, you can see which areas of perimenopause are affecting your life the most. Keep a journal or track your symptoms as you progress through the book to see how dietary and lifestyle adjustments impact your well-being over time.

Setting personalised health goals

Setting achievable, personalised goals can help you approach perimenopause with a sense of purpose. These goals should be realistic and focus on enhancing your quality of life rather than achieving perfection.
For example:

- **If energy management is your main goal**: Focus on including nutrient-dense foods, adopting a consistent sleep routine, and incorporating gentle exercise that boosts vitality.
- **If stabilising weight is a priority**: Concentrate on balanced meals with lean proteins, fibre, and healthy fats, while monitoring portion sizes and reducing processed sugars.
- **If you're struggling with mood swings**: Prioritise omega-3-rich foods, such as salmon and walnuts, magnesium-rich leafy greens, and mindfulness practices that promote calm and stability.

Breaking these goals down into small, manageable actions will make them easier to integrate into your daily life.
For instance, if better sleep is a goal, you might start by setting a consistent bedtime

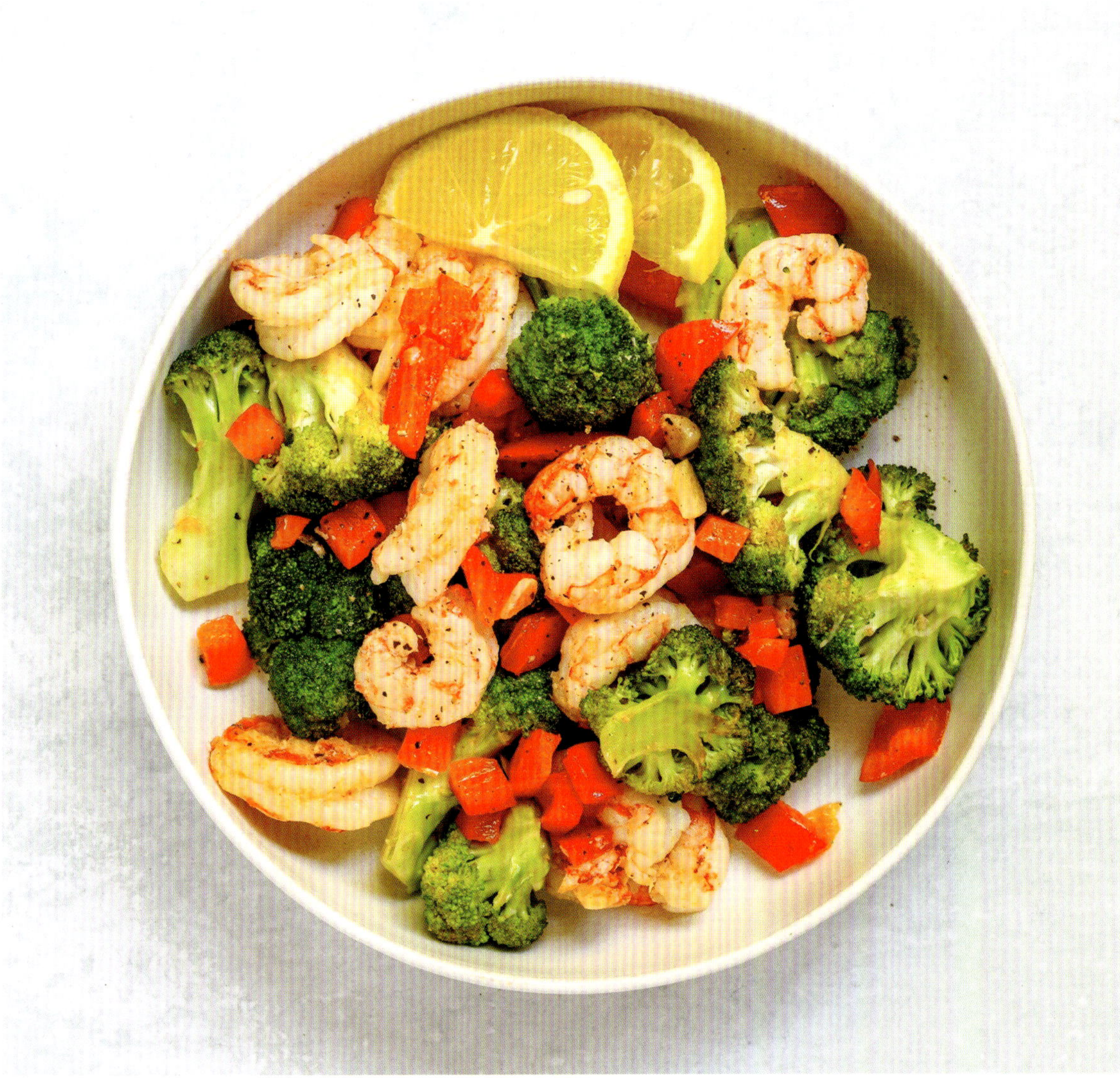

and incorporating magnesium-rich foods like spinach, almonds, and pumpkin seeds into your diet. Each small step brings you closer to a balanced, healthy, and fulfilling approach to perimenopause.

Setting goals in this way allows you to tune into your body's needs while also keeping you feeling motivated to make positive changes. These personalised health goals are a foundation for the chapters to come, guiding you as you explore the nutritional and lifestyle strategies that best support your unique experience of perimenopause.

CHAPTER 2

ESSENTIAL NUTRIENTS FOR THE PERIMENOPAUSAL BODY

Managing perimenopause means taking extra care with your diet. Each nutrient you consume has a unique impact on your physical and mental health, especially as hormonal changes affect everything from energy levels and mood to bone health and metabolism. By focusing on a balanced diet that meets the unique needs of perimenopause, you can greatly reduce common symptoms and boost your sense of well-being. Here, I'll guide you through the essential macronutrients, vitamins, and minerals that can help you feel more balanced, energised, and prepared for the journey ahead.

Balancing macronutrients

Macronutrients – proteins, fats, and carbohydrates – are foundational for a balanced diet that supports physical health, mental clarity, and stable energy. Each macronutrient plays a vital role in managing perimenopausal symptoms, making it crucial to understand how to incorporate them in ways that best support you.

- **Proteins:**
  Protein is essential for building and maintaining muscle mass, which becomes increasingly important as estrogen levels drop. Estrogen helps preserve lean muscle and supports a healthy metabolism, so when levels decrease, muscle mass can diminish, making it harder to keep weight stable. By eating lean proteins – such as chicken, fish, tofu, eggs, and legumes – you can help stabilise blood sugar, reduce cravings, and maintain lean muscle. Protein is also highly satiating, meaning it can help you feel full for longer periods and prevent energy dips between meals. For perimenopausal women, aiming for 60 grams of protein per day can provide benefits for muscle maintenance and blood sugar stability.

  Adding protein-rich snacks, like a handful of almonds or a boiled egg, can also be an effective way to curb cravings and keep energy levels stable throughout the day. If you're incorporating strength exercises, protein becomes even more essential, as it helps repair muscle and supports recovery. Protein requirements vary based on factors like age, activity level, and health goals, but a good general guideline is 1–1.5 grams of protein per kilogram of body weight per day. For instance, a 70kg woman going through perimenopause would need between 70–105 grams of protein daily.

- **Healthy fats**:
  Fat is often misunderstood, but healthy fats are crucial for brain health, hormone production, and reducing inflammation in the body. Fatty acids, especially omega-3s found in foods like salmon, chia seeds, flaxseeds, and walnuts, are known to support cognitive function and may even alleviate symptoms like mood swings and anxiety. Omega-3s have anti-inflammatory properties that help reduce the body's stress response, which can be particularly helpful for managing perimenopausal symptoms.

  Healthy fats also promote the absorption of fat-soluble vitamins like vitamins A, D, E, and K, which are essential for skin, bone, and immune health. Incorporating avocados, olive oil, nuts, and seeds into your meals is a great way to ensure you're getting these benefits. I recommend aiming for a small portion of healthy fats with each meal – whether it's a sprinkle of seeds on your salad, a spoonful of olive oil on roasted vegetables, or a slice of avocado with breakfast. Not only will it help you feel more satisfied, but it also provides crucial nutrients to support your overall well-being.

- **Complex carbohydrates**:
  Carbohydrates are an important part of any diet, but the type of carbs you choose can make a big difference in how you feel. Complex carbohydrates – found in whole grains like oats, quinoa, brown rice, and starchy vegetables like sweet potatoes – provide a slow, steady release of energy and are high in fibre. Fibre is especially important during perimenopause because it helps stabilise blood sugar levels, supports digestion, and promotes a feeling of fullness.

  Unlike simple carbohydrates, which can cause quick spikes in blood sugar followed by crashes, complex carbohydrates provide sustained energy, reducing the likelihood of cravings and mood swings. Whole grains also contain B vitamins, which are essential for energy production and cognitive health. Aiming for a balance of complex carbohydrates in your diet can prevent the energy crashes often experienced during perimenopause, allowing you to feel steady and focused throughout the day.

  When building your meals, aim for a balanced plate: include a lean protein, a healthy fat, and a portion of complex carbohydrates, along with a generous serving of vegetables. This combination of macronutrients will keep you satiated, energised, and mentally sharp. Creating meals with this balance also helps manage symptoms like fatigue, cravings, and irritability, making it easier to feel your best each day.

Vital vitamins and minerals

While macronutrients form the structure of a balanced diet, vitamins and minerals are the powerhouses that support various bodily functions, from bone health and muscle maintenance to mood regulation. During perimenopause, certain vitamins and minerals become particularly important for symptom management and overall health.

- **Calcium and Vitamin D**:
  One of estrogen's roles is to aid calcium absorption, so as estrogen levels drop, the risk of bone density loss increases. This makes calcium and vitamin D essential for maintaining strong bones. Calcium-rich foods like leafy green vegetables, dairy products, almonds, and fortified plant-based milk can support bone health. However, without adequate vitamin D, calcium can't be absorbed properly. Since vitamin D is primarily obtained through sunlight exposure, many people find it beneficial to include vitamin D-rich foods, like fatty fish, eggs, and fortified products. If sunlight exposure is limited, a vitamin D supplement may be helpful. Together, calcium and vitamin D help you protect bone density, allowing you to stay active, reduce the risk of fractures, and maintain a strong, healthy body as you age.

- **Magnesium**:
  Magnesium is often called the "relaxation mineral" because of its ability to reduce anxiety, improve sleep quality, and support muscle relaxation. During perimenopause, magnesium's role becomes even more significant, as it helps manage stress and improves sleep, which are common challenges during this phase. Foods like spinach, pumpkin seeds, almonds, and whole grains are excellent sources of magnesium and can be easily incorporated into your meals. Magnesium also supports heart health and muscle function, making it a valuable addition to any diet. If you struggle with restless sleep or frequent muscle cramps, you may find that magnesium-rich foods or a magnesium supplement can make a noticeable difference in how you feel.

- **B Vitamins**:
  B vitamins, including B6, B12, and folate, play a crucial role in energy production, brain health, and mood stabilisation. Found in foods like eggs, leafy greens, whole grains, and lean meats, these vitamins are especially important during perimenopause, as they help combat fatigue and "brain fog." B vitamins support the nervous system, making them particularly helpful in managing symptoms of anxiety or irritability. If you're feeling mentally or physically drained, adding B vitamin-rich foods to your meals can provide a much-needed boost, helping you maintain energy and focus throughout the day. For some women, a B-complex supplement may be beneficial, but always consult with your healthcare provider before adding new supplements.

Adding these key vitamins and minerals to your diet can be transformative for your perimenopausal journey. By prioritising nutrient-dense foods, you're not only addressing immediate symptoms but also setting up a foundation for long-term health and vitality.

Managing sugar and caffeine

Sugar and caffeine are often quick fixes for low energy or cravings, but they can have a significant impact on perimenopausal symptoms. While occasional indulgences are normal, keeping an eye on your sugar and caffeine intake can help you feel more balanced, energised, and calm.

- **Reducing sugar**:
  Excess sugar can lead to blood sugar spikes and crashes, causing sudden shifts in energy and mood. This roller-coaster effect can make symptoms like fatigue and irritability worse, and it may even contribute to weight gain, particularly around the abdomen. Reducing added sugars in your diet – such as those in sweets, soft drinks, and processed foods – can prevent these energy crashes and keep your mood stable. Opt for natural sugars found in fruits, which come paired with fibre to slow down the release of sugar into your bloodstream. By focusing on whole foods, you not only lower your sugar intake but also boost your intake of vitamins, minerals, and antioxidants that support overall health.
- **Managing caffeine**:
  Many of us turn to caffeine for a quick energy boost, but too much caffeine can worsen symptoms of perimenopause, such as anxiety, irritability, and disrupted sleep. High caffeine intake, especially in the afternoon, can interfere with sleep quality, leading to a cycle of fatigue and stress. If you're sensitive to caffeine, consider gradually reducing your intake or switching to herbal teas or green tea, which offer a gentler lift without the post-caffeine crash. Green tea, for instance, contains a compound called L-theanine, which promotes calmness while providing an energy boost, making it a suitable alternative during perimenopause.

Managing sugar and caffeine doesn't mean you need to eliminate them entirely, but reducing their presence in your daily routine can lead to more consistent energy levels and improved mood. Small adjustments in these areas can make a noticeable difference in how you feel, helping you to stay energised and steady throughout the day.

CHAPTER 3

THE PERIMENOPAUSE MEAL PLAN

A well-designed meal plan can be a game-changer during perimenopause, helping you address symptoms, stabilise weight, and maintain energy levels throughout the day. This four-week meal plan is carefully crafted with nutrient-dense foods to support your body's needs during this phase. Each meal is balanced to provide essential macronutrients, vitamins, and minerals that play a role in managing perimenopausal symptoms, promoting mental clarity, and ensuring stable energy. The meal plan also includes flexibility for dietary preferences and provides practical advice on portion sizes and meal timing to make this journey as simple and enjoyable as possible.

Monthly meal plan

My monthly perimenopause meal plan is designed to address the common challenges of perimenopause, including fluctuating energy, weight gain, mood swings, and fatigue. Each week includes a balanced selection of meals high in fibre, lean proteins, healthy fats, and antioxidants, all of which work together to nourish your body and stabilise hormonal shifts. The goal is to create a sustainable, nourishing diet that not only supports physical health but also promotes mental and emotional well-being.

Incorporating a variety of ingredients ensures you're getting the nutrients needed to support hormonal balance, boost energy, and prevent common perimenopausal symptoms. By following this meal plan, you'll establish a foundation for long-term health that goes beyond perimenopause, supporting a healthy transition into menopause and beyond.

Each day's meal structure has been designed to deliver balanced nutrients that support hormonal health, stabilise blood sugar levels, and reduce perimenopausal symptoms. Every meal should ideally include a mix of:

- **Lean proteins**: Options like chicken, fish, beans, or tofu are excellent sources of protein to support muscle maintenance and curb cravings. Protein also helps regulate blood sugar levels, preventing energy dips and mood swings.
- **Healthy fats**: Avocados, nuts, seeds, and olive oil are sources of healthy fats that support hormone production and brain health. Including healthy fats with each meal can help you feel full and satisfied while promoting stable energy.

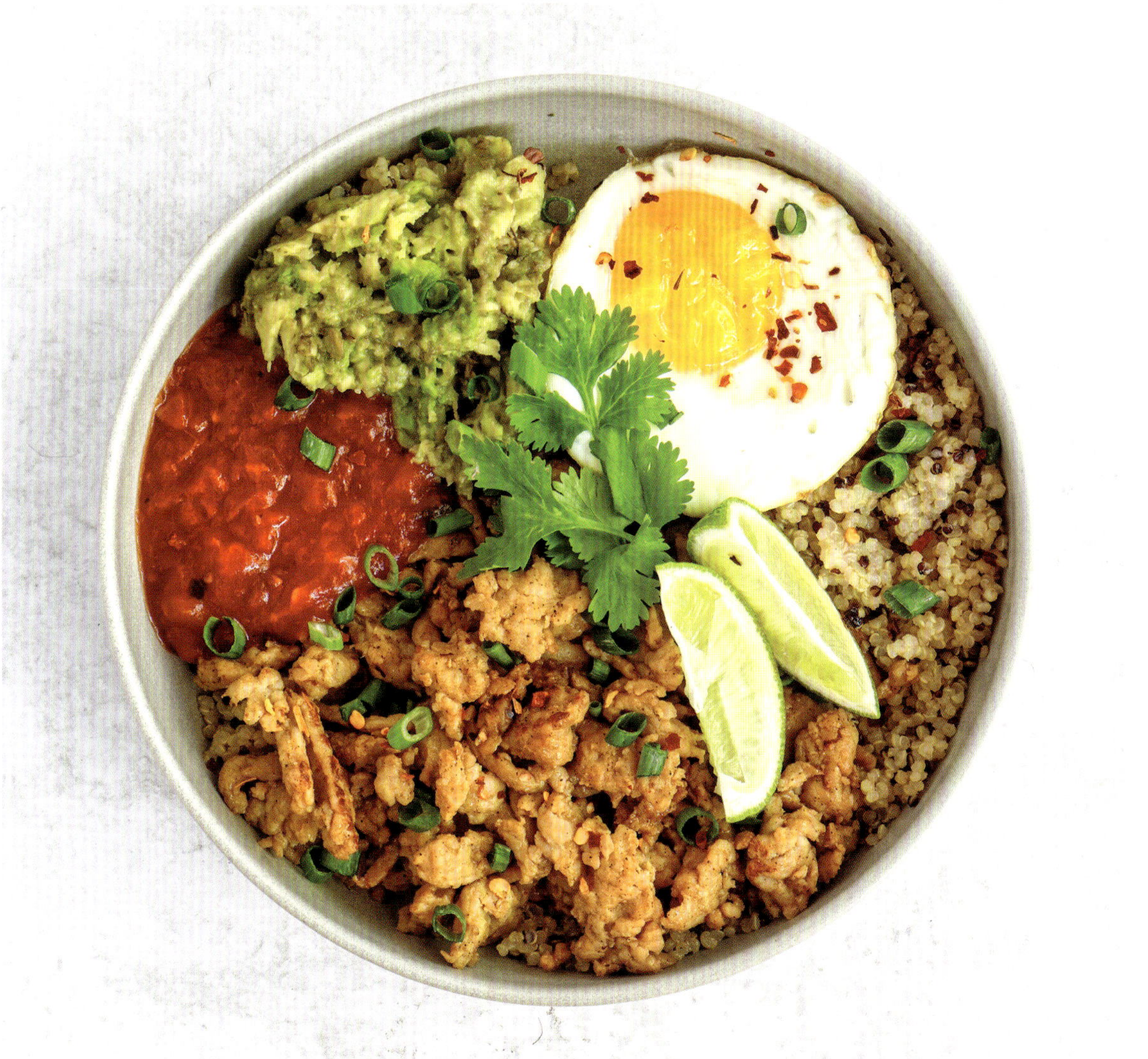

- **High-fibre carbohydrates**: Complex carbs like quinoa, oats, leafy greens, and sweet potatoes provide a steady source of energy and support digestion. These carbs help prevent the blood sugar spikes and crashes that can contribute to fatigue and irritability.

By including these elements in each meal, you're nourishing your body in a way that promotes mental clarity, boosts energy, and supports stable hormone levels. This structure can help make each day more predictable and enjoyable, allowing you to focus on other aspects of your life rather than worrying about how to manage your diet.

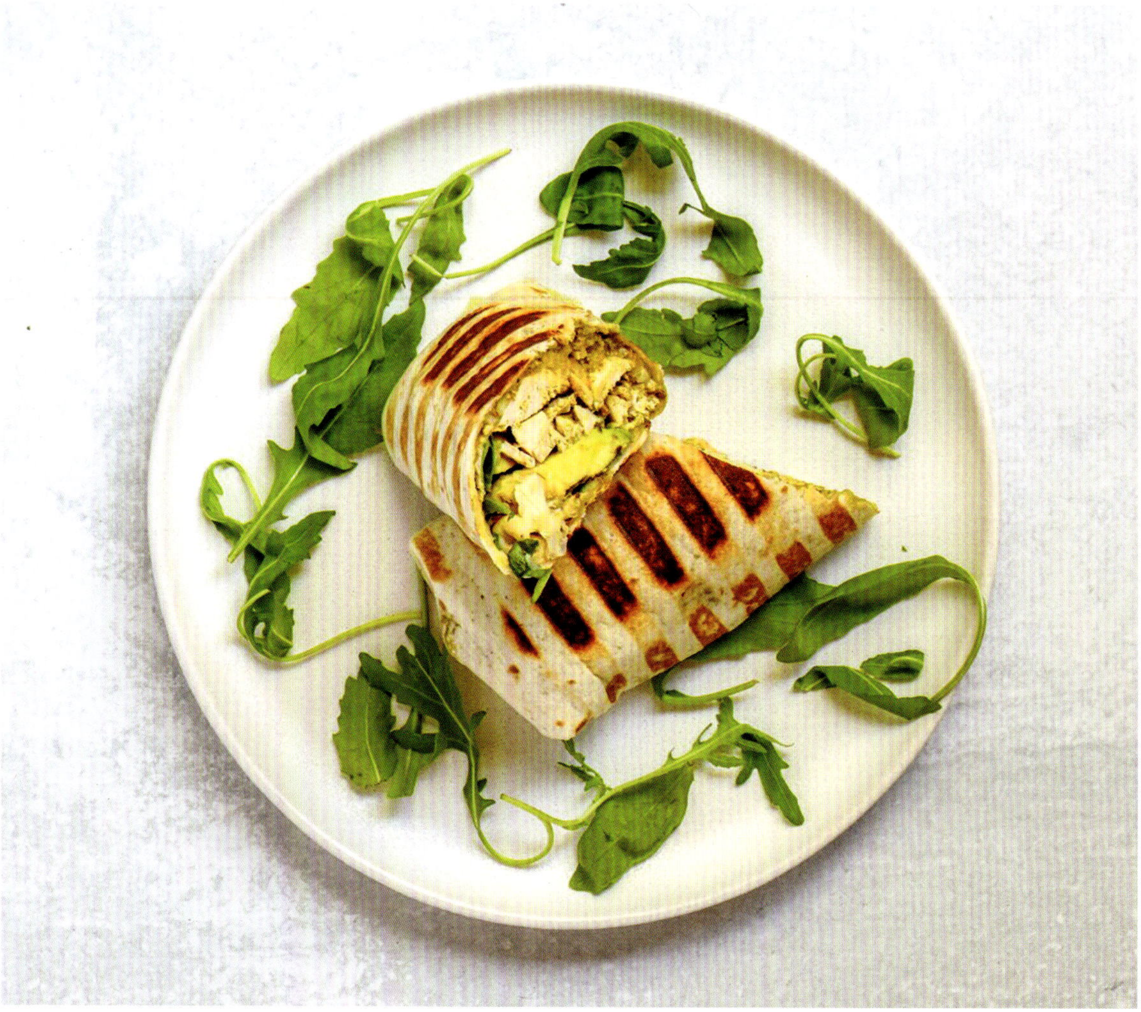

Flexibility
A flexible meal plan is a sustainable one, so each meal plan includes options for substitutions and snack alternatives. Whether you're vegetarian, gluten-free, or simply looking for variety, the plan offers suggestions for alternative ingredients and meal ideas that fit your preferences. Here's how you can tailor the meal plan to suit your needs:

- **Vegetarian or plant-based options**: Substitute animal-based proteins with plant-based options like tofu, tempeh, chickpeas, and lentils. These are not only rich in protein but also offer fibre and essential vitamins that support perimenopausal health.
- **Gluten-free adjustments**: If you're following a gluten-free diet, grains like quinoa, brown rice, and sweet potatoes

can be excellent alternatives to wheat-based carbohydrates.

- **Dairy-free choices**: Swap dairy products with plant-based options like almond or coconut milk, and choose dairy-free yoghurt made from coconut or almond for a creamy, satisfying snack.

The flexibility of this plan also extends to snacks. For those who need a mid-morning or afternoon boost and don't have time to make one of my recipes included in the plan, snacks like nuts, Greek yoghurt, apple slices with almond butter, or vegetable sticks with hummus can be nutritious and satisfying. The key is to listen to your body's needs, and if a particular meal or snack doesn't resonate, feel free to swap it with a similar option that fits your preferences.

Portion and timing guidelines

Portion control and meal timing are key to maintaining steady energy levels, reducing cravings, and managing symptoms effectively. Here are some practical tips to help you manage portions and timing:

- **Portion control**: Aim for portions that leave you feeling satisfied but not overly full. A balanced meal might include a palm-sized portion of protein, a fist-sized portion of complex carbohydrates, a thumb-sized portion of healthy fats, and plenty of non-starchy vegetables. These portion sizes provide enough energy to sustain you without overloading your body, making it easier to maintain a stable weight.
- **Meal timing**: Eating meals at regular intervals can prevent blood sugar dips and spikes, which are often accompanied by fatigue and cravings. Aim for three balanced meals each day, with a small snack or two if needed. For example, try eating breakfast within an hour of waking up, followed by lunch about four to five hours later, and dinner by early evening. Avoid skipping meals, as this can lead to blood sugar imbalances and intensified cravings later on.
- **Snack timing**: If you find that your energy wanes between meals, a small snack can help stabilise blood sugar. Mid-morning and mid-afternoon snacks work well for many people. Choose snacks that are balanced, like a handful of nuts with fruit or Greek yoghurt with a sprinkle of flaxseeds.

By following these portion and timing guidelines, you'll help your body maintain balanced energy levels and prevent the crashes and cravings that can make perimenopause symptoms more challenging. Regular meal timing and portion control can also improve mood, reduce irritability, and support consistent energy levels, making it easier to manage daily tasks and enjoy life.

CHAPTER 4

MEAL PLANS

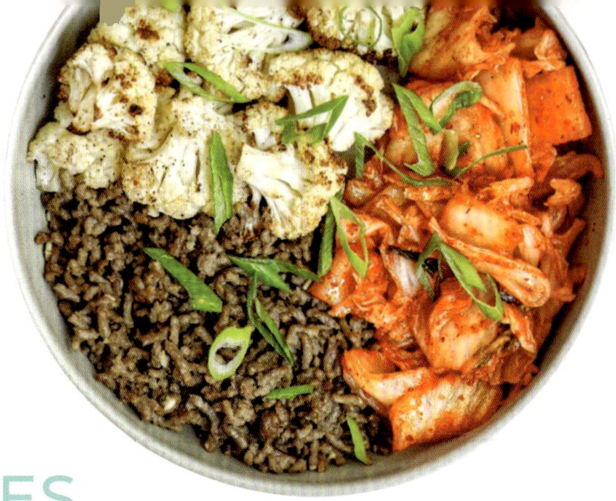

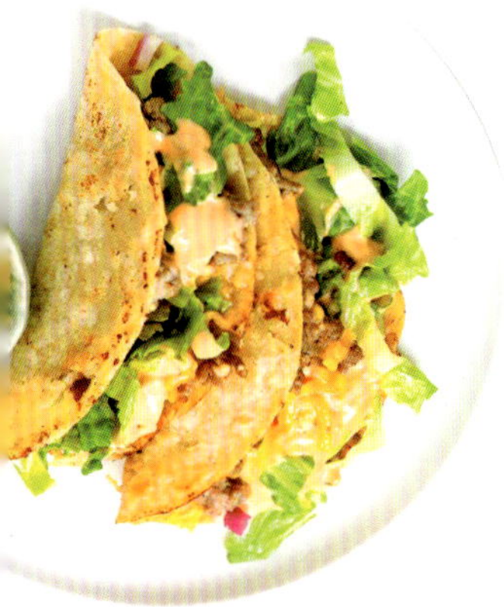

RECIPES
WEEK 1

PESTO CHICKPEA TOAST
TEX-MEX BREAKFAST BOWL
SPICY CHICKEN BREAKFAST WRAP
COTTAGE CHEESE BANANA BREAD
ONE POT PARMESAN CHICKEN
KIMCHI BEEF CAULIFLOWER BOWL
GARLIC BUTTER CHICKEN & ASPARAGUS
TAHINI CHICKEN SALAD
COCONUT SHRIMP WITH RICE
PEANUT CHICKEN WITH COCONUT RICE
TERIYAKI SALMON BOWL
AIR FRYER KOREAN PORK LETTUCE WRAPS
BLUEBERRY TAHINI PROTEIN SMOOTHIE
PROTEIN ALMOND DONUTS
BEETROOT CHOCOLATE BROWNIES

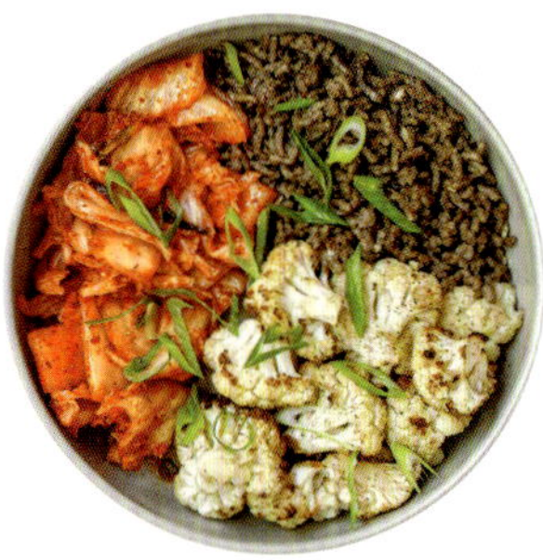

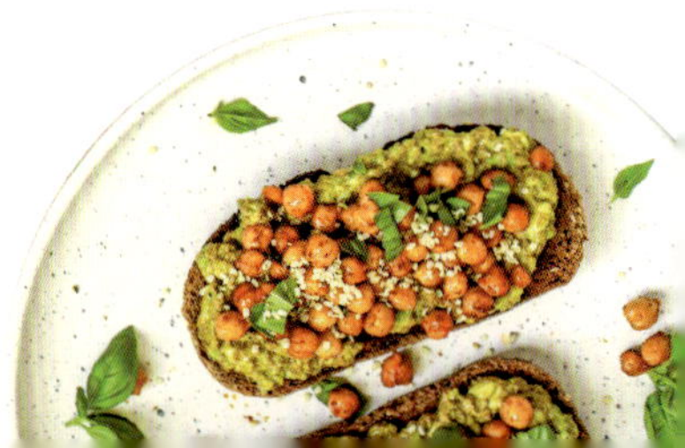

WEEKLY SHOPPING LIST

PRODUCE

3 avocados
4 bananas
4 lemons
2 limes
blueberries
red grapes
1 red onion
2 bunches green onions (spring onions)
2 bulbs garlic root
ginger
celery
2 cucumbers
1 tomato
2 heads lettuce spinach
asparagus
small head cauliflower
edamame beans
cooked beetroot
basil
cilantro (coriander)
dill
parsley
dried golden raisins
frozen green peas (garden peas)

PROTEIN

1.3 lb (570 g) boneless, skinless chicken thighs
3.5 lb (1.6kg) boneless, skinless chicken breast
1 lb (450 g) shredded roast chicken
1 lb (450 g) ground turkey (turkey mince)
12 oz (340 g) 95% lean ground beef (beef mince)
1 lb (450 g) pork tenderloin
1 lb (450 g) shrimp (prawn)
1.5 lb (680 g) salmon fillet
8 eggs unsweetened almond milk
natural yogurt
butter
cottage cheese
Parmesan cheese

DRY GOODS

basmati rice
Jasmine rice
almond meal (ground almonds)
coconut flakes
hazelnuts
peanuts
pecans
hemp hearts
hemp seeds
quinoa
sesame seeds
all purpose flour
baking powder
baking soda
unsweetened cocoa powder
vanilla extract
sprinkles
black pepper
red pepper flakes (chili flakes)
paprika
garlic powder
onion powder ground
cinnamon
Chinese five spice
taco seasoning
dried oregano
Herbes de Provence

STAPLES & MISC

coconut oil
sesame oil
brown sugar
coconut sugar
honey
maple syrup
3.5 oz. (100 g) can chickpeas
14 oz. (400 g) can full fat coconut milk
chicken broth (stock)
white wine vinegar
rice wine vinegar
tamari sauce
sriracha sauce
gochujang (Korean chili paste, or use similar)
tahini
Dijon mustard
pesto
salsa
adobo sauce
hot sauce
kimchi
applesauce (apple purée)
vanilla protein powder
wholemeal bread
flour tortilla wraps
panko breadcrumbs
70% dark chocolate

PANTRY STAPLES

You should have five basic essentials for these recipes in your kitchen. They're used so frequently that they're not included in the weekly ingredient shopping list.

These staples are **vegetable oils** like **olive oil** for cooking and **extra virgin olive oil** for dressing; a variety of **vinegar** (white and red wine vinegar, apple cider vinegar) for adding acidity and balancing flavours in marinades; sauces, and condiments; **salt** (sea or Himalayan salt); and **black pepper** for seasoning.

Sample Weekly Meal Planner

	BREAKFAST	LUNCH
Monday	TEX-MEX BREAKFAST BOWL	KIMCHI BEEF CAULIFLOWER BOWL
Tueday	TEX-MEX BREAKFAST BOWL	KIMCHI BEEF CAULIFLOWER BOWL
Wednesday	SPICY CHICKEN BREAKFAST WRAP	TAHINI CHICKEN SALAD
Thursday	SPICY CHICKEN BREAKFAST WRAP	TAHINI CHICKEN SALAD
Friday	BLUEBERRY TAHINI PROTEIN SMOOTHIE	GARLIC BUTTER CHICKEN & ASPARAGUS
Saturday	PESTO CHICKPEA TOAST	GARLIC BUTTER CHICKEN & ASPARAGUS
Sunday	COTTAGE CHEESE BANANA BREAD	ONE POT PARMESAN CHICKEN

SNACK	DINNER
PROTEIN ALMOND DONUTS	COCONUT SHRIMP WITH RICE
PROTEIN ALMOND DONUTS	PEANUT CHICKEN WITH COCONUT RICE
BEETROOT CHOCOLATE BROWNIES	PEANUT CHICKEN WITH COCONUT RICE
BEETROOT CHOCOLATE BROWNIES	ONE POT PARMESAN CHICKEN
COTTAGE CHEESE BANANA BREAD	TERIYAKI SALMON BOWL
COTTAGE CHEESE BANANA BREAD	MEAL OUT – ENJOY!
BLUEBERRY TAHINI PROTEIN SMOOTHIE	AIR FRYER KOREAN PORK LETTUCE WRAPS

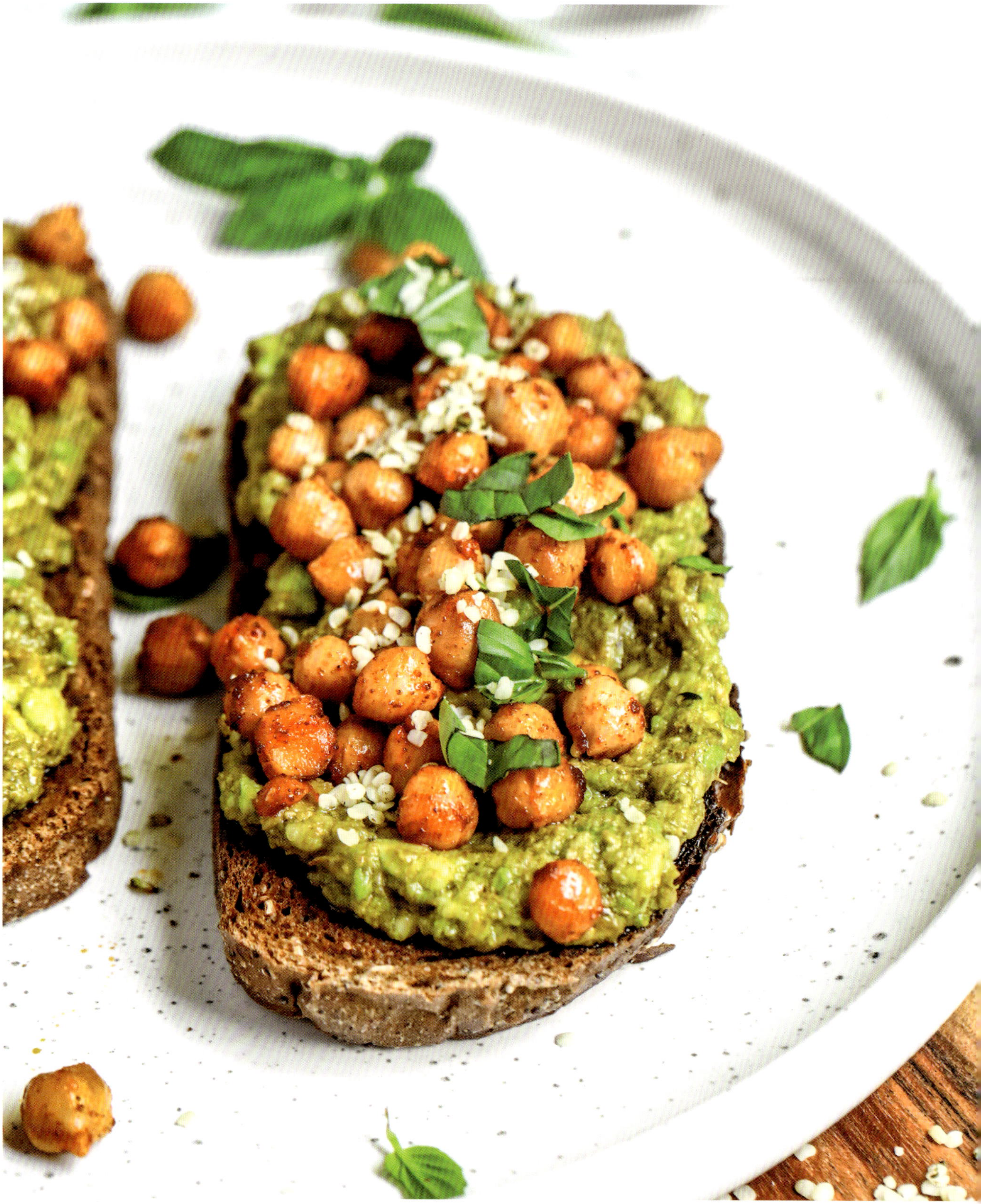

SERVES **2** | **20** MINUTES

PESTO CHICKPEA **TOAST**

INGREDIENTS

3.5 oz (100 g) **canned chickpeas**, drained
1 tsp **paprika**
2 slices **wholemeal bread**, toasted
3 tbsp **pesto**
1 tbsp **basil**, chopped, to garnish
1 tbsp **hemp seeds**, to garnish

METHOD

- Preheat the oven to 425°F (220°C). Prepare a baking tray lined with baking paper.
- Place the drained chickpeas on the baking tray, season with paprika, salt and pepper, drizzle with olive oil and toss well to coat. Roast in the oven for 15 minutes.
- Toast the bread and spread pesto evenly. Top with the roasted chickpeas and garnish the toasts with basil and hemp seeds.

ENERGY: **385** Kcal	CARBS: **35** g	PROTEIN: **14** g	FAT: **21** g

SERVES **4** | **15** MINUTES

TEX-MEX BREAKFAST BOWL

INGREDIENTS

3.2 oz (90 g) **dry quinoa**
1 lb (450 g) **lean ground turkey**
1 oz (30 g) **taco seasoning**
4 **eggs**
1 **avocado**, mashed
4 tbsp **salsa**
1 **green onion**, sliced
1 tbsp **cilantro**, chopped
lime wedges, to serve

METHOD

- Cook the quinoa according to package instructions.
- Heat 1 tsp olive oil in a non-stick skillet over medium heat and add the ground turkey and taco seasoning. Mix to combine and sauté until the turkey is cooked all the way through, then remove from the skillet and set aside. In the same skillet, fry the eggs until done to your liking.
- Assemble the breakfast bowls by dividing the cooked quinoa, turkey and mashed avocado equally between 4 bowls. Top each bowl with a tablespoon of salsa and a fried egg, then garnish with green onions and cilantro. Serve immediately with lime wedges.

STORAGE

- The cooked turkey and quinoa can be stored in individual containers in the refrigerator until you are ready to assemble the bowls, making it perfect for meal prep.

ENERGY: **448** Kcal | CARBS: **25** g | PROTEIN: **33** g | FAT: **24** g

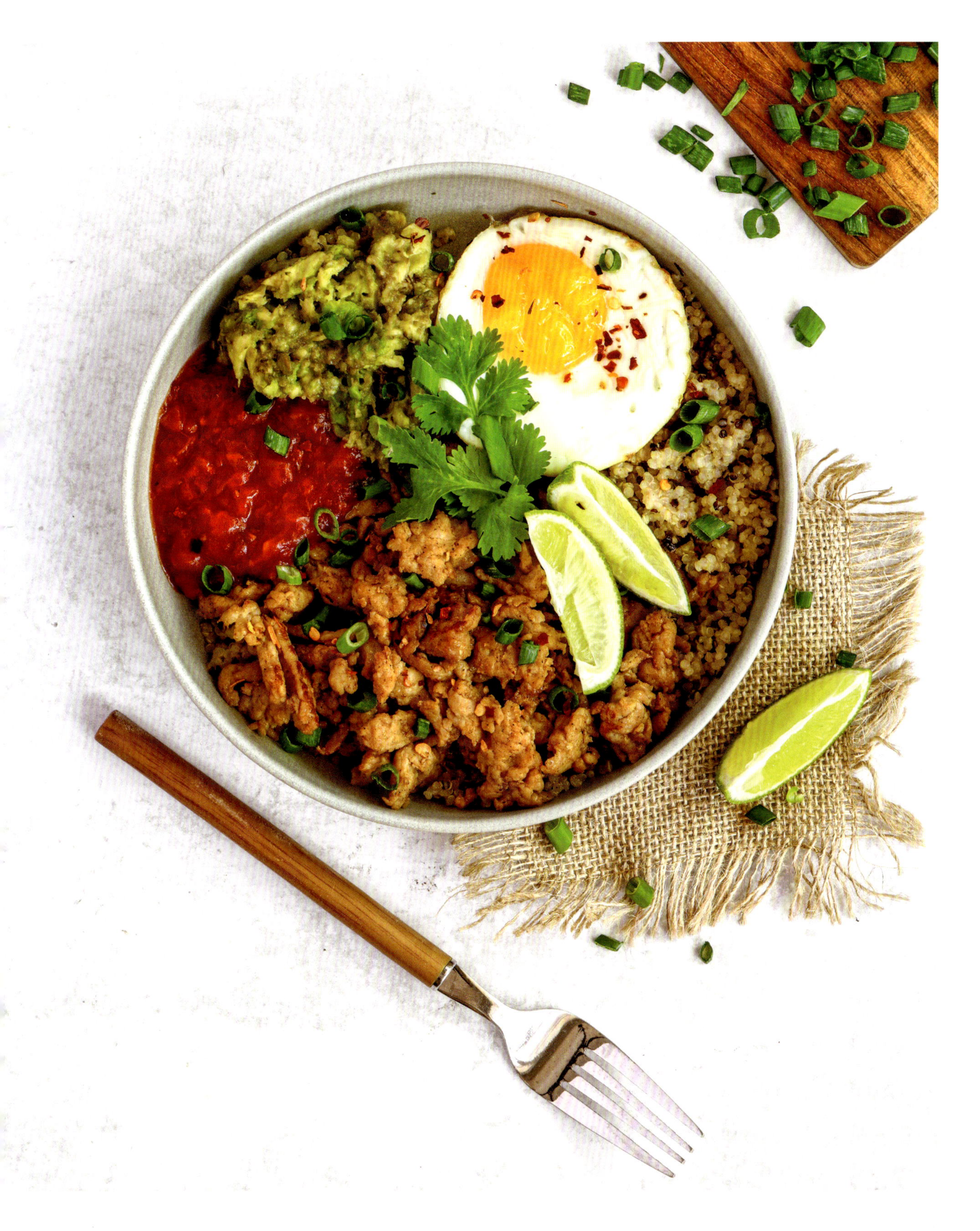

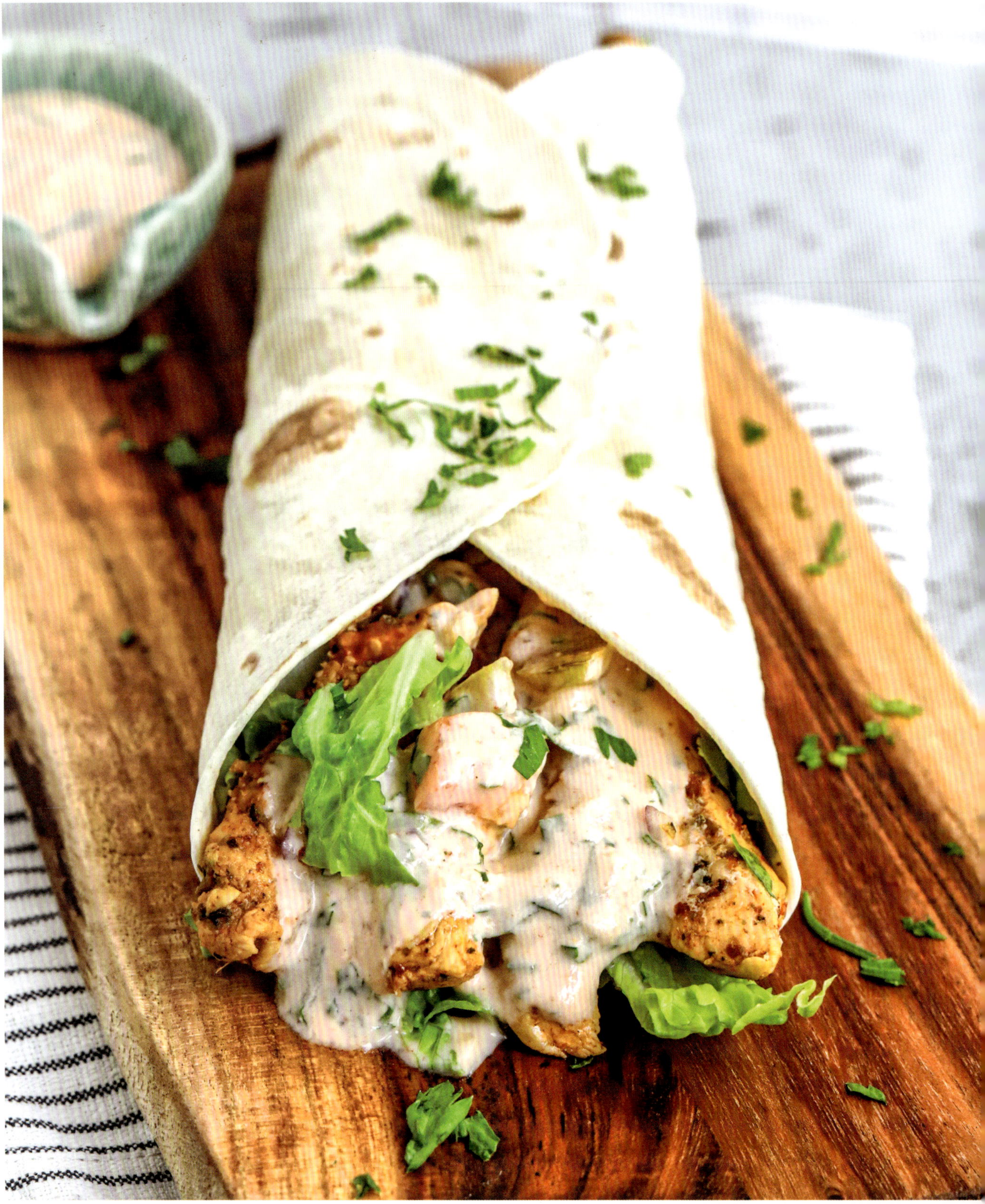

SERVES **4** | **18** MINUTES

SPICY CHICKEN BREAKFAST WRAP

INGREDIENTS

1 lb (450 g) **chicken breast**
4 **flour tortilla wraps**
2.6 oz (70 g) **lettuce**, shredded
½ **red onion**, chopped
1 **tomato**, chopped

Spices and seasoning

2 **garlic** cloves, minced
1 tbsp **dried oregano**
1 tbsp **paprika**
1 tsp **onion powder**
1 tsp **red pepper flakes**
1 **lemon**, juiced

For the spicy sauce

3.5 oz (100 g) **natural yogurt**
1 tbsp **hot sauce**
1 **clove garlic**, minced
1 tbsp **parsley**, chopped
splash **lemon juice**, to taste

METHOD

- Slice the chicken breasts into strips, place into a large bowl, along with all the spices and seasoning, 1 tsp salt and pepper, and stir to combine. Add the lemon juice and mix well until the chicken changes colour.
- Place the chicken into a large non-stick skillet and cook over medium heat for 8 minutes until golden brown and cooked through.
- While the chicken is cooking, make the spicy sauce by adding all the sauce ingredients into a bowl, season with salt and pepper to taste, and mix until well combined.
- To assemble the wrap, place the shredded lettuce on the wrap, then add the grilled chicken, red onion and tomatoes. Top with spicy sauce, then wrap and enjoy.

ENERGY: **312** Kcal	CARBS: **27** g	PROTEIN: **33** g	FAT: **8** g

SERVES **12** | **65** MINUTES

COTTAGE CHEESE BANANA BREAD

INGREDIENTS

3 **bananas**, mashed
3.2 oz (90 g) **coconut sugar**
2.7 oz (90 ml) **coconut oil**, melted
2 **eggs**
5.3 oz (150 g) **cottage cheese**
4 tbsp **hemp hearts**
1 tsp **vanilla extract**
7.4 oz (210 g) **all-purpose flour**
1 tsp **baking soda**
1 tsp **ground cinnamon**
2 tbsp **pecans**, chopped

METHOD

- Preheat the oven to 325°F (160°C). Grease a loaf pan with nonstick baking spray or use a silicone pan.
- Place the mashed bananas in a large bowl, add the sugar and oil and stir to combine. Add the eggs, cottage cheese, hemp hearts and vanilla extract and mix again.
- To that same bowl add the flour, baking soda, cinnamon and ½ tsp of salt. Fold the dry ingredients into the wet until just combined.
- Transfer the batter into the prepared loaf pan. Top with the pecan nuts and bake in the oven for 55–60 minutes, until a toothpick entered into the centre comes out clean.
- Remove from the oven and set aside to cool for 15 minutes, then remove from the pan and place on a wire rack to cool before slicing and serving.

ENERGY: **235** Kcal	CARBS: **29** g	PROTEIN: **5** g	FAT: **11** g

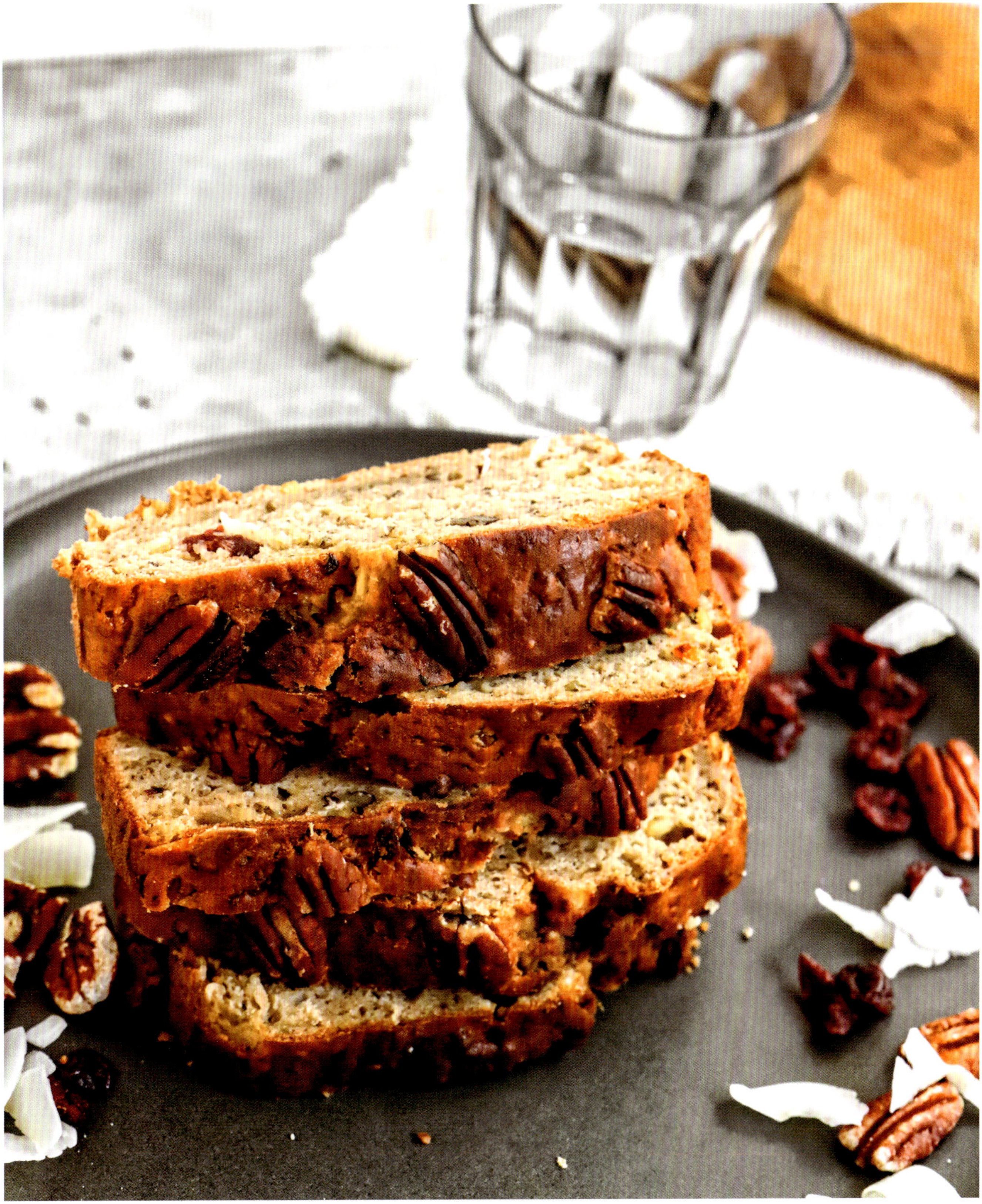

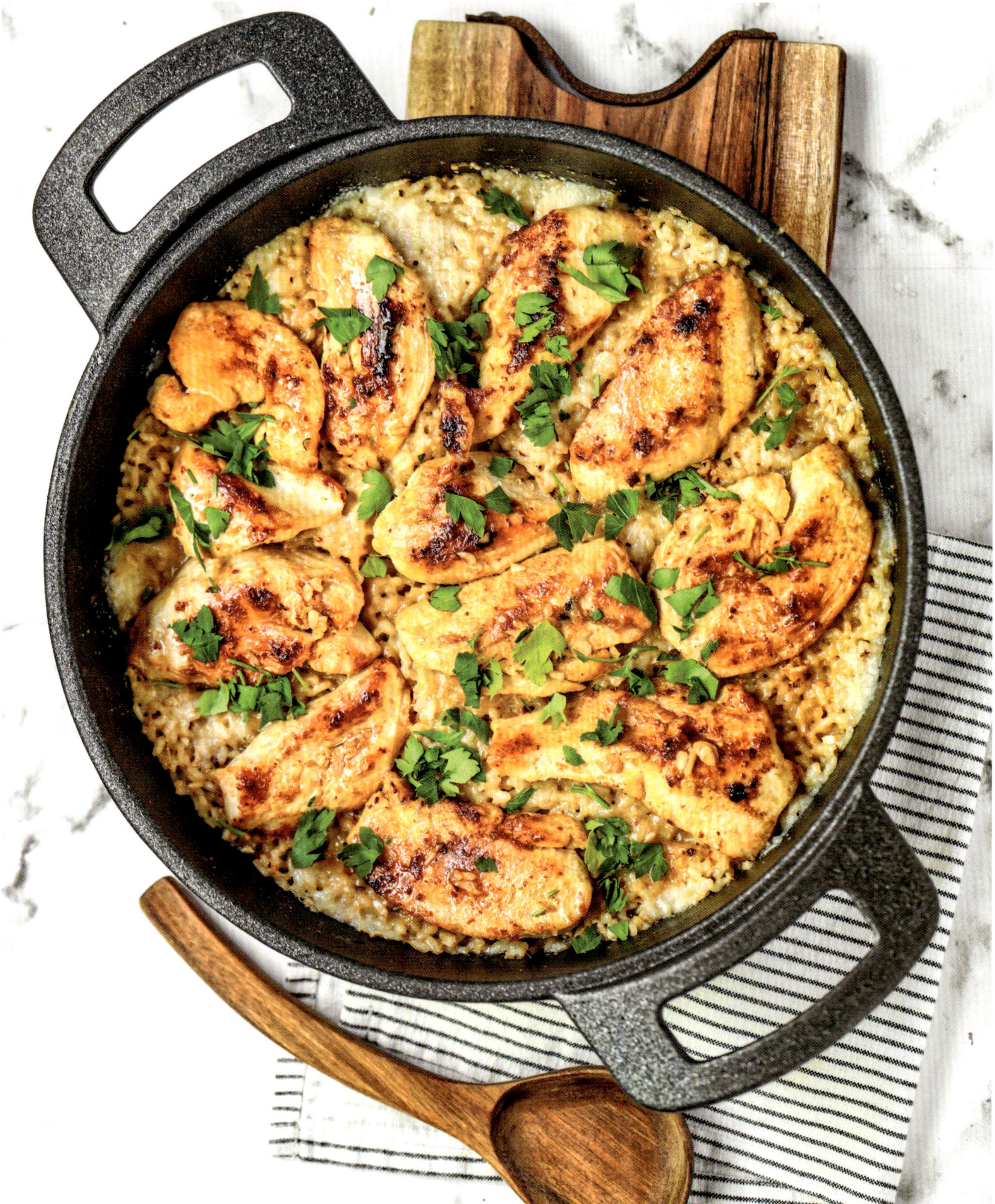

SERVES **4** | **35** MINUTES

ONE POT PARMESAN CHICKEN

INGREDIENTS

1.1 lb (500 g) **chicken breast**, cut in half
½ tsp **garlic powder**
2 tbsp **butter**
1 cloves **garlic**
pinch of **red pepper** flakes
7 oz (200 g) **basmati rice**
1.3 pints (720 ml) **chicken broth**
1.6 oz (45 g) **Parmesan cheese**, grated
1 tbsp **parsley**, chopped

METHOD

- Season the chicken with salt, pepper and garlic powder.
- Heat 2 tbsp olive oil in a large non-stick skillet and fry the chicken for 8 minutes until golden on both sides. Remove the chicken from the skillet and set aside.
- Using the same skillet, melt the butter, add the garlic and red pepper flakes, and cook for 1–2 minutes. Then add the rice, chicken broth and stir to combine, then bring to a boil. Cover with a lid and cook over medium heat for around 10 minutes.
- Remove the lid and stir the rice, then top with the Parmesan cheese. Now arrange the chicken fillets on top and cook over a low heat for 5 minutes. Garnish with freshly chopped parsley and serve.

ENERGY: **496** Kcal | CARBS: **42** g | PROTEIN: **37** g | FAT: **20** g

SERVES **2** | **40** MINUTES

KIMCHI BEEF CAULIFLOWER BOWL

INGREDIENTS

1 small **cauliflower**, florets
1 tsp **Chinese five spice**
12 oz (340 g) **95% lean ground beef**
1 **clove garlic**, minced
½ tsp **root ginger**, minced
6 tbsp **kimchi**
1 **green onion**, sliced

METHOD

- Preheat the oven to 400°F (200°C). Line a baking sheet with baking paper.
- Add the cauliflower, Chinese five spice, 1 tbsp of olive oil, salt and pepper into a large bowl. Toss to combine, then spread over the prepared baking sheet. Roast the cauliflower in the oven for 20–25 minutes, or until browned.
- Meanwhile, heat 1 tbsp of olive oil in a pan over medium heat. Add the ground beef, garlic and ginger, and season with salt and pepper. Cook the beef for 5–7 minutes, breaking it up as it cooks, until it is cooked through.
- Divide the cauliflower, beef and kimchi equally between 2 bowls and garnish with the sliced green onion. Serve immediately.

ENERGY: **449** Kcal | CARBS: **16** g | PROTEIN: **40** g | FAT: **25** g

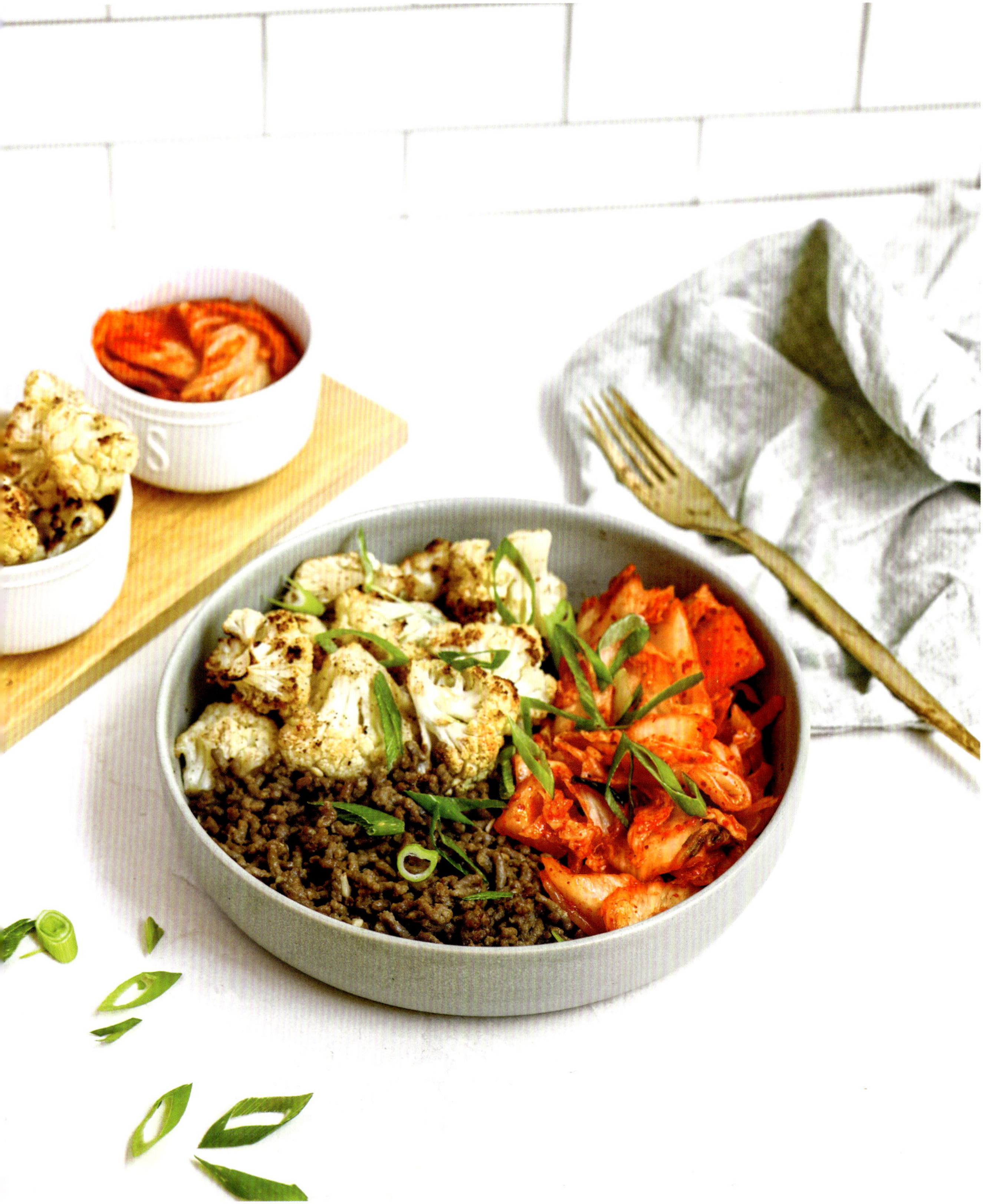

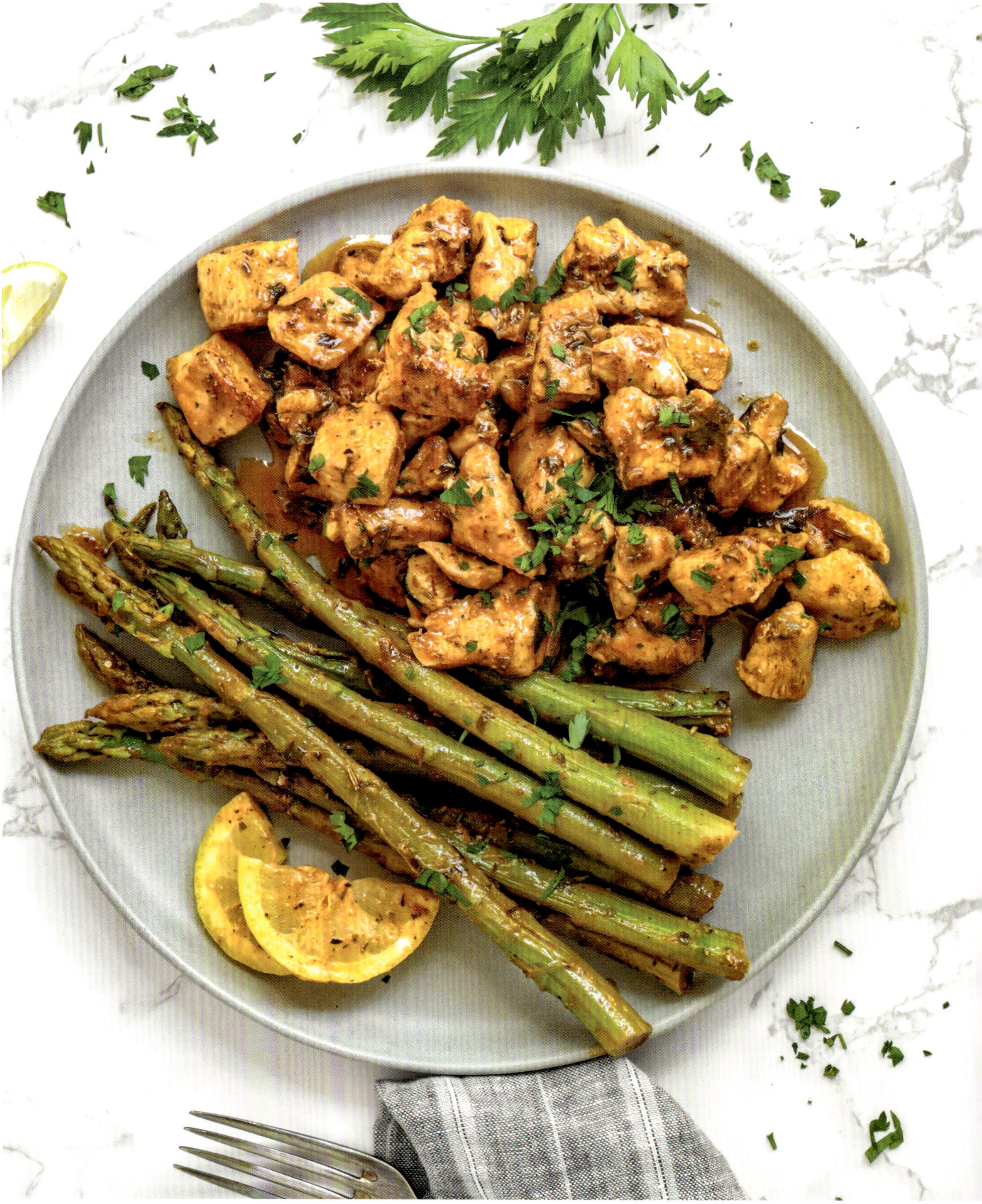

SERVES **4** | **30** MINUTES

GARLIC BUTTER CHICKEN AND ASPARAGUS

INGREDIENTS

1.4 lb (650 g) **chicken breasts**, diced
2 tsp **onion powder**
8.8 oz (250 g) **asparagus**, trimmed
4 tbsp **butter**, divided
2 cloves **garlic**, minced, divided
1 tsp **Herbes de Provence**
4.2 fl oz (125 ml) **chicken broth**
juice of ½ **lemon**
1 tbsp **hot sauce**
1 tbsp **parsley**, chopped

METHOD

- Season the chicken with salt, pepper and onion powder.
- Blanch the asparagus in boiling water for 2 minutes, then drain and soak in ice cold water. Drain again and set aside.
- Melt 2 tbsp of butter with the olive oil in a large skillet over medium heat. Cook the chicken until golden brown. Lower the temperature and add 1 minced garlic clove and the herbs. Stir and cook for 1 more minute, then remove from the skillet and set aside.
- In the same skillet over medium-high heat, add the remaining garlic, then deglaze the skillet with chicken broth. Bring to a simmer and allow to reduce the liquid to half. Add the remaining 2 tbsp of butter, lemon juice, hot sauce and parsley, and stir to combine.
- Add the asparagus and warm through for 2 minutes. Push the asparagus to the side, add the sautéed chicken back to the pan, and stir for a further minute to reheat. Serve immediately.
- **Serving suggestion:** garnish with more parsley, chili flakes and lemon slices.

ENERGY: **325** Kcal | CARBS: **4** g | PROTEIN: **39** g | FAT: **17** g

TAHINI CHICKEN SALAD

INGREDIENTS

1 lb (450 g) **chicken breast**, cooked, shredded
3.5 oz (100 g) **celery**, diced
2.6 oz (75 g) **red grapes**, halved
0.5 oz (12 g) **parsley**, chopped
2.3 oz (65 g) **hazelnuts**, chopped
1.4 oz (40 g) **golden raisins**, chopped

For the tahini dill sauce

2 oz (60 g) **tahini**
4 tbsp **lemon juice**
4 tbsp **white wine vinegar**
2 tbsp **fresh dill**
1 tbsp **Dijon mustard**
½ tbsp **adobo sauce**

METHOD

- Place all the salad ingredients in a bowl, and stir to combine. Add all the sauce ingredients in a jar, season with salt and 1 tsp of black pepper, and mix well.
- Add the sauce to the salad ingredients and mix until everything is evenly coated in the sauce. If required, adjust the seasoning, and serve.

ENERGY: 434 Kcal | CARBS: 19 g | PROTEIN: 40 g | FAT: 22 g

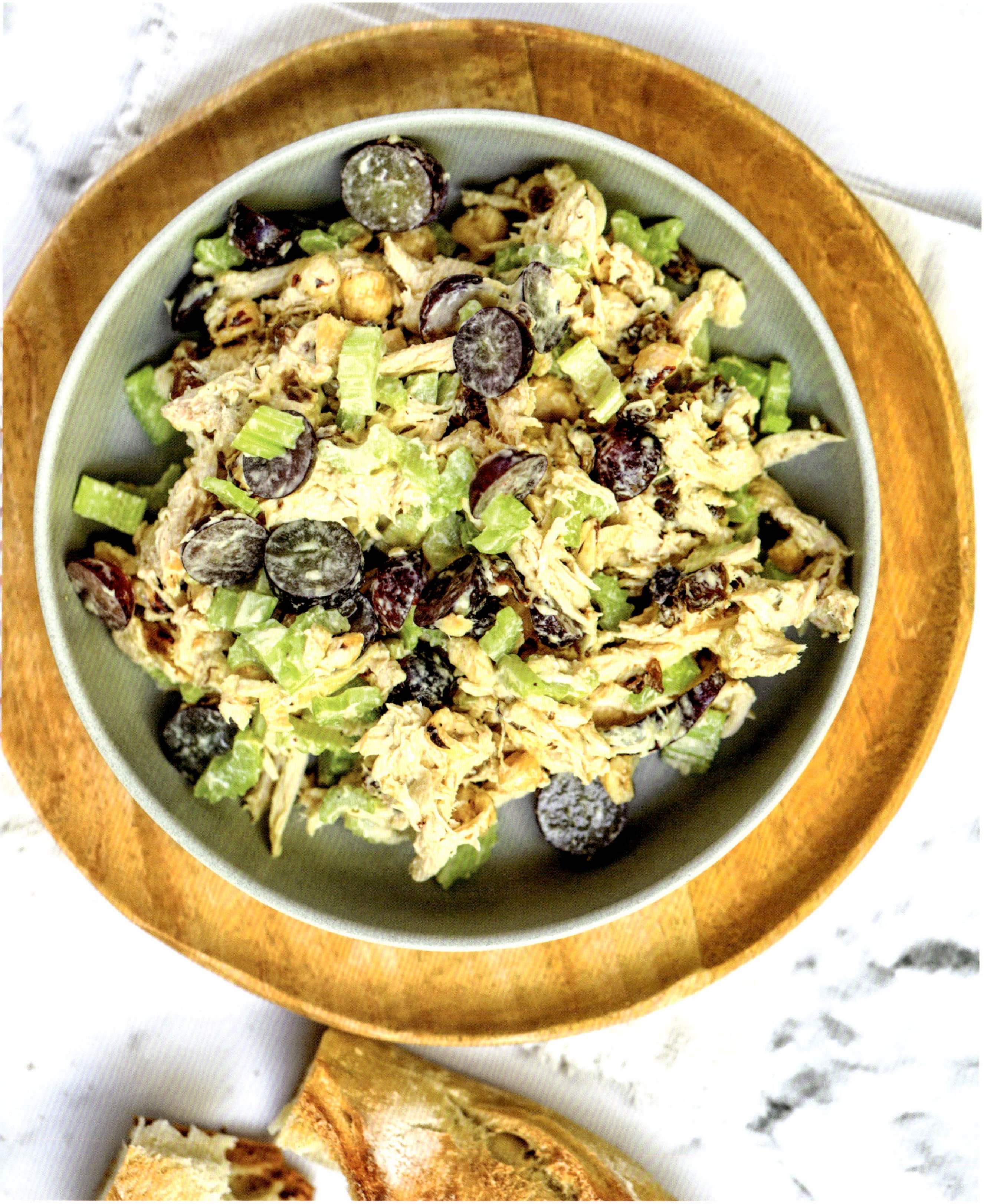

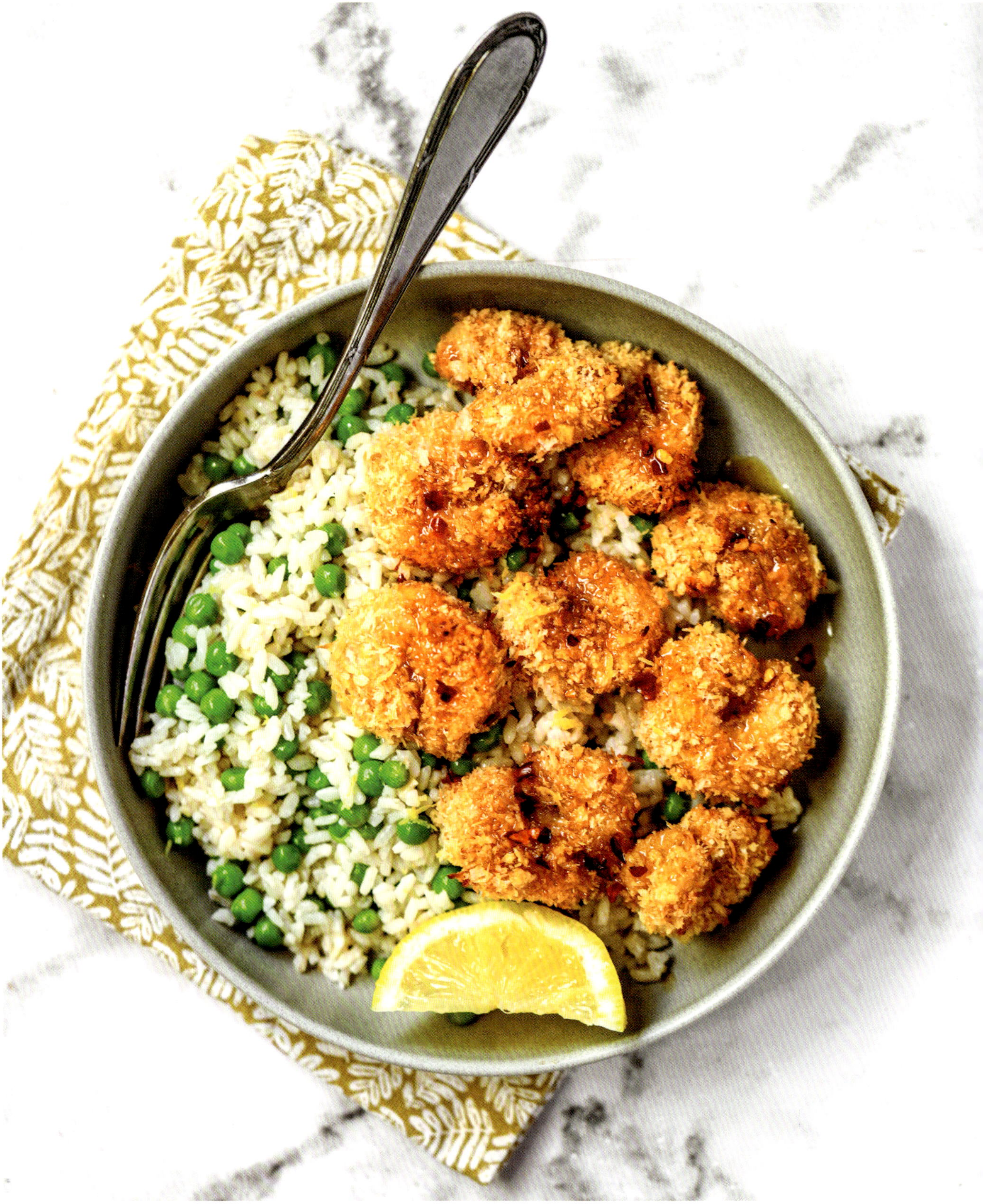

SERVES **4** | **20** MINUTES

CRISPY COCONUT SHRIMP WITH RICE

INGREDIENTS

For the coconut shrimp

2 oz (60 g) **panko breadcrumbs**
2 oz (60 g) **unsweetened coconut flakes**
2 oz (60 g) **all-purpose flour**
½ tsp **paprika**
2 **eggs**, beaten
1 lb (450 g) **shrimp**, thawed, tails removed

For the rice

7.4 oz (210 g) **Jasmine rice**
10 oz (280 g) **green peas**
juice and zest of 1 **lemon**
handful of **fresh herbs** or **leafy greens**
1 **clove garlic**, minced
2 tbsp **butter**

For the butter honey sauce

4 tbsp melted **butter**
2 tbsp **honey**
1 tbsp **Dijon mustard**

METHOD

- Cook the rice according to instructions on the packaging. Preheat the oven to 325°F (160°C).
- Place the panko breadcrumbs and coconut flakes on a baking sheet, and toast in the oven for 10 minutes, stirring occasionally, until golden. Remove from the oven and raise the oven temperature to 425°F (210°C).
- Prepare 3 bowls, combine flour, paprika, and ½ tsp salt in the first; egg in the second, and the toasted panko/coconut mixture in the third.
- Coat each shrimp first in the flour, then the egg, then press into the panko/coconut mixture. Place the coated shrimp back on the baking sheet and spray or drizzle with some olive oil. Bake in the oven for 10 minutes.
- Meanwhile, finish the rice. Add the green peas, lemon juice and zest, the fresh herbs or leafy greens (depending on preference), garlic, and butter into the hot rice and mix to combine. Make a sauce by mixing the melted butter with the honey and Dijon mustard in a small bowl. Serve the shrimps over the rice with a generous drizzle of sauce.

ENERGY: **498** Kcal | CARBS: **60** g | PROTEIN: **24** g | FAT: **18** g

SERVES **4** | **25** MINUTES

PEANUT CHICKEN WITH COCONUT RICE

INGREDIENTS

For the ginger peanut chicken

1.3 lb (570 g) **boneless, skinless chicken thighs**, cut into bite-sized pieces
1-inch (2.5 cm) piece of **ginger**, grated
3 **green onions**, thinly sliced (white parts and green parts separated)
zest and juice of 1–2 **limes**
2 tbsp **brown sugar**
2–3 cloves **garlic**, minced
2 oz (60 g) **roasted peanuts**, chopped
0.5 oz (10 g) **cilantro**, chopped
1 oz (30 g) **spinach** (or **bok choy**)

For the coconut rice

7.5 oz (210 g) **jasmine rice**
12 fl oz (360 ml) **water**
14 oz (400 g) can **full-fat coconut milk**

METHOD

- In a bowl, mix the chicken thighs with the ginger, green onions (white parts only), lime zest, brown sugar, 1½ tsp salt, and 1 tbsp olive oil. Cover the bowl and set aside to marinate for 20 minutes (or up to 2 hours if time allows).
- To make the coconut rice, add the rice, water, coconut milk and a pinch os salt to a large pot, and stir to combine. Place the pot over a medium-high heat, and bring to a boil, before turning to low and simmering the rice until cooked.
- Heat a large non-stick skillet over medium-high heat, add the marinated chicken and cook until the chicken starts to caramelize. Once the chicken is cooked through, turn the heat down, add the garlic and peanuts and sauté for 5 minutes.
- Now stir through the cilantro, remaining green onion and spinach. Squeeze the lime juice into the skillet and check the seasoning, adding more salt and pepper if required.
- Serve the chicken over the coconut rice. Garnish with more green onions, chopped peanuts and cilantro (optional).

ENERGY: **688** Kcal	CARBS: **58** g	PROTEIN: **37** g	FAT: **32** g

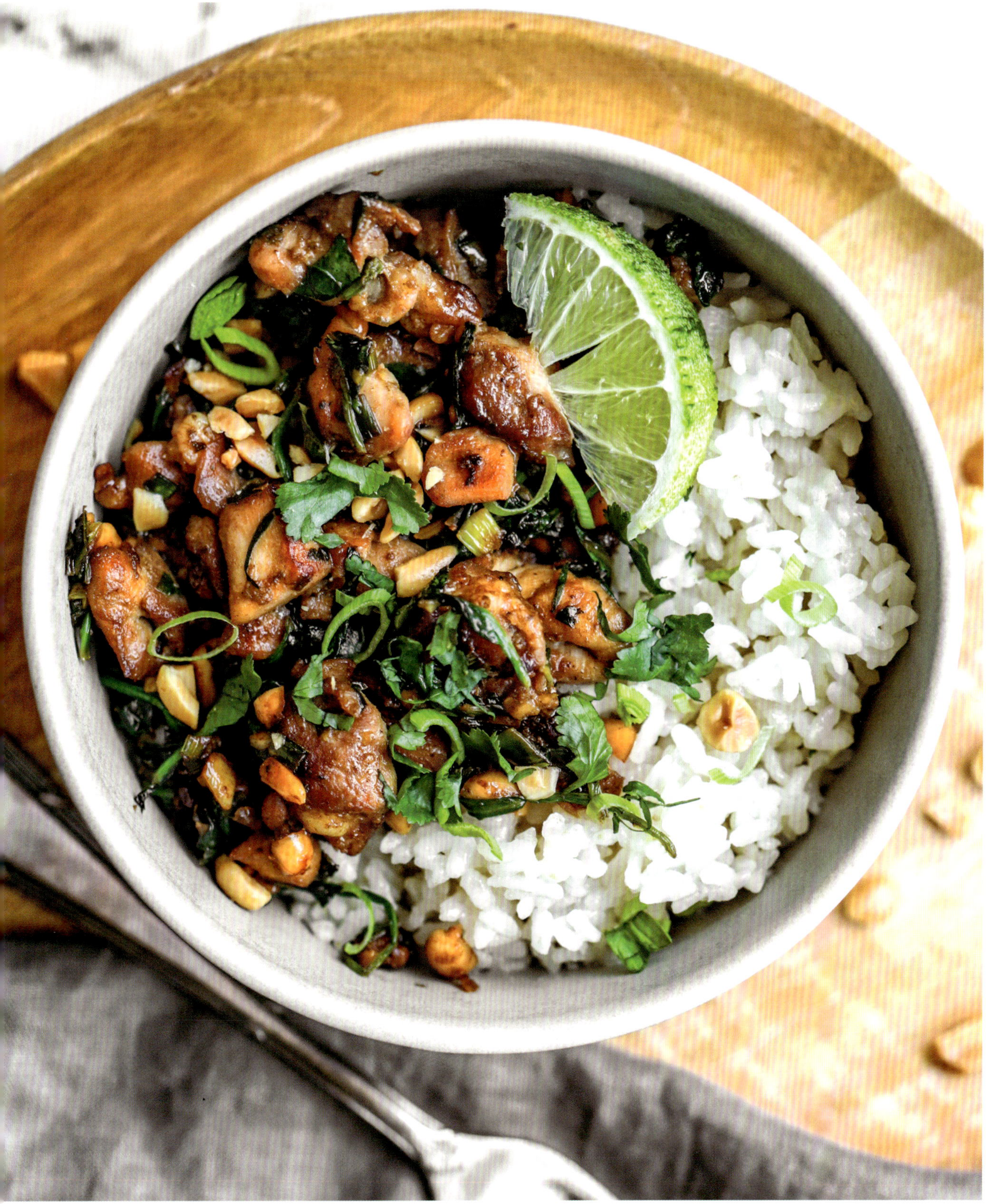

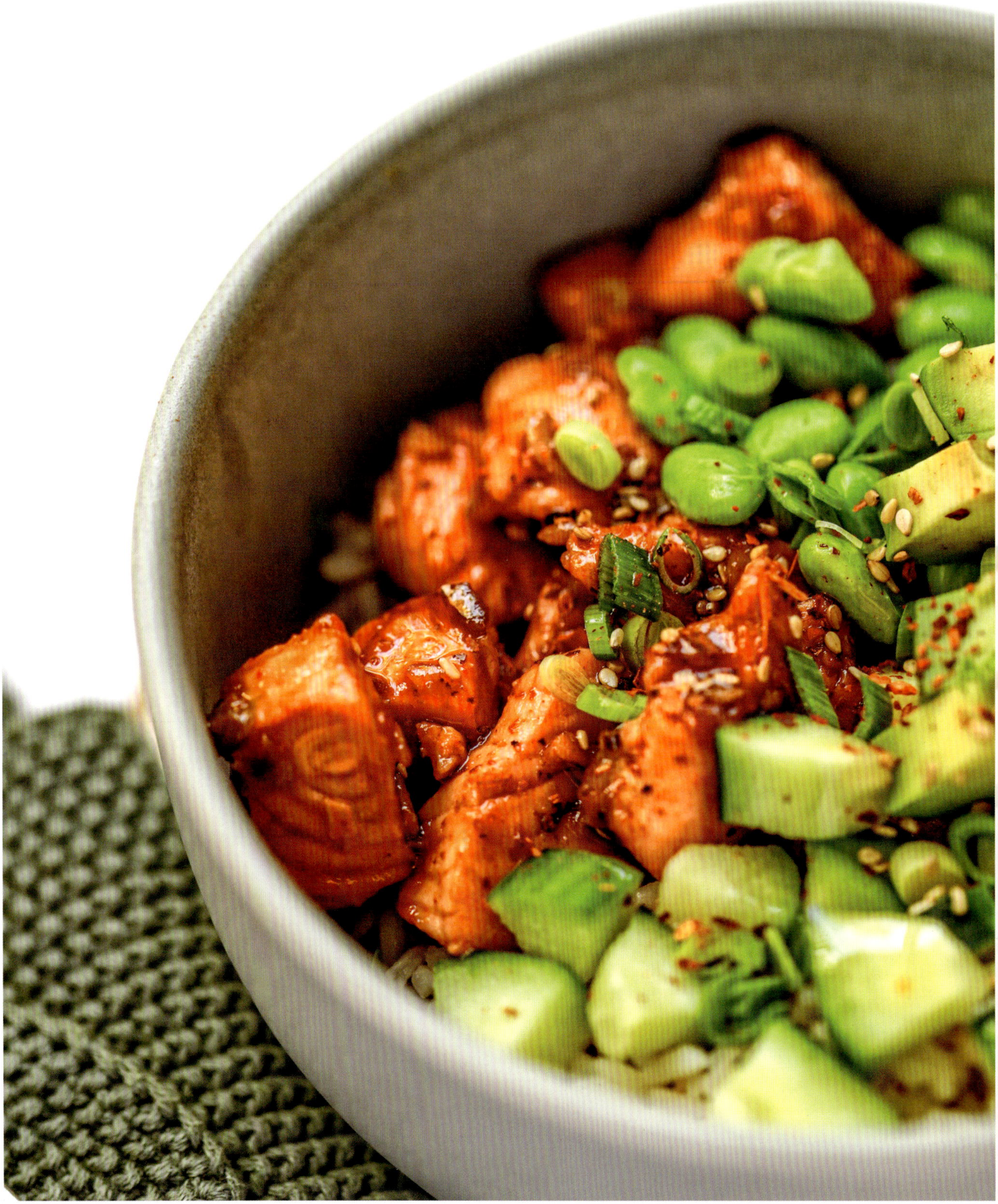

SERVES **6** | **20** MINUTES

TERIYAKI SALMON BOWL

INGREDIENTS

12.7 oz (360 g) cooked **basmati rice**
6 tbsp **rice wine vinegar**
2 tbsp **maple syrup**, divided
2 tbsp **sesame seeds**, divided
1 tbsp **tamari sauce**
2 tsp **sesame oil**
1 tsp **sriracha sauce**
½ tsp fresh **ginger**, grated
½ tsp fresh **garlic**, grated
1.5 lb (680 g) **salmon fillet**, skinned, cubed
5.6 oz (160 g) **edamame beans**
3.5 oz (100 g) **cucumber**, sliced
2 **avocados**, sliced
1 oz (30 g) **green onions**, minced
chili flakes, to garnish

METHOD

- Add the cooked basmati rice to a large bowl. In a separate small bowl, whisk the rice vinegar, 1 tbsp of maple syrup and 1 tsp salt. Pour the vinegar mixture into the rice, add 1 tbsp of sesame seeds, and mix well to combine.
- In a small bowl, make the teriyaki sauce by combining the remaining tbsp of maple syrup with the tamari, sesame oil, sriracha, ginger and garlic.
- Heat a large skillet over medium heat and add 1 tbsp of olive oil. Add the salmon chucks and cook for a minute on each side. Now add the teriyaki sauce, bring the heat up to high and toss the salmon in the sauce until well coated. Continue cooking for another 5 minutes, then remove from the heat.
- Divide the sesame rice into 6 bowls and top with the edamame beans, cucumber and avocado slices. Now add the teriyaki salmon to each of the bowls and top with additional sauce from the pan. Lastly, top each bowl with green onions, the remaining sesame seeds, and chili flakes and serve immediately.

ENERGY: **470** Kcal	CARBS: **35** g	PROTEIN: **33** g	FAT: **22** g

SERVES **4** | **40** MINUTES

AIR FRYER KOREAN PORK LETTUCE WRAPS

INGREDIENTS

1 lb (450 g) **pork tenderloin**
2 oz (60 g) **gochujang (Korean chili paste)**
1 **clove garlic**, finely grated
2 tbsp **honey**
1 tbsp **toasted sesame oil**
¼ tsp fresh **ginger**, finely grated
1 head **lettuce**, leaves separated
1 **cucumber**, sliced
4 **green onions**, sliced
6.5 oz (185 g) **cooked rice**, for serving

METHOD

- Cut the pork tenderloin in half crosswise and season with salt.
- Place the gochujang, garlic, honey, sesame oil, and ginger into a medium bowl and stir to combine. Transfer a ¼ cup of the gochujang mixture to a small bowl and stir in the rice wine vinegar; and set this bowl aside for serving.
- Add the pork tenderloin to the bowl with the remaining sauce and toss to coat.
- Lightly coat an air-fryer basket with cooking spray. Place the pork in the basket and cook at 350°F (180°C) for 17–20 minutes, turning occasionally, until the pork is golden brown. Remove the pork from the air fryer and set it aside to rest for 10 minutes before slicing.
- Place the slices of pork in the lettuce leaves, along with the cucumber, green onions and cooked rice. Serve with the small bowl of reserved sauce alongside.

ENERGY: **294** Kcal	CARBS: **34** g	PROTEIN: **26** g	FAT: **6** g

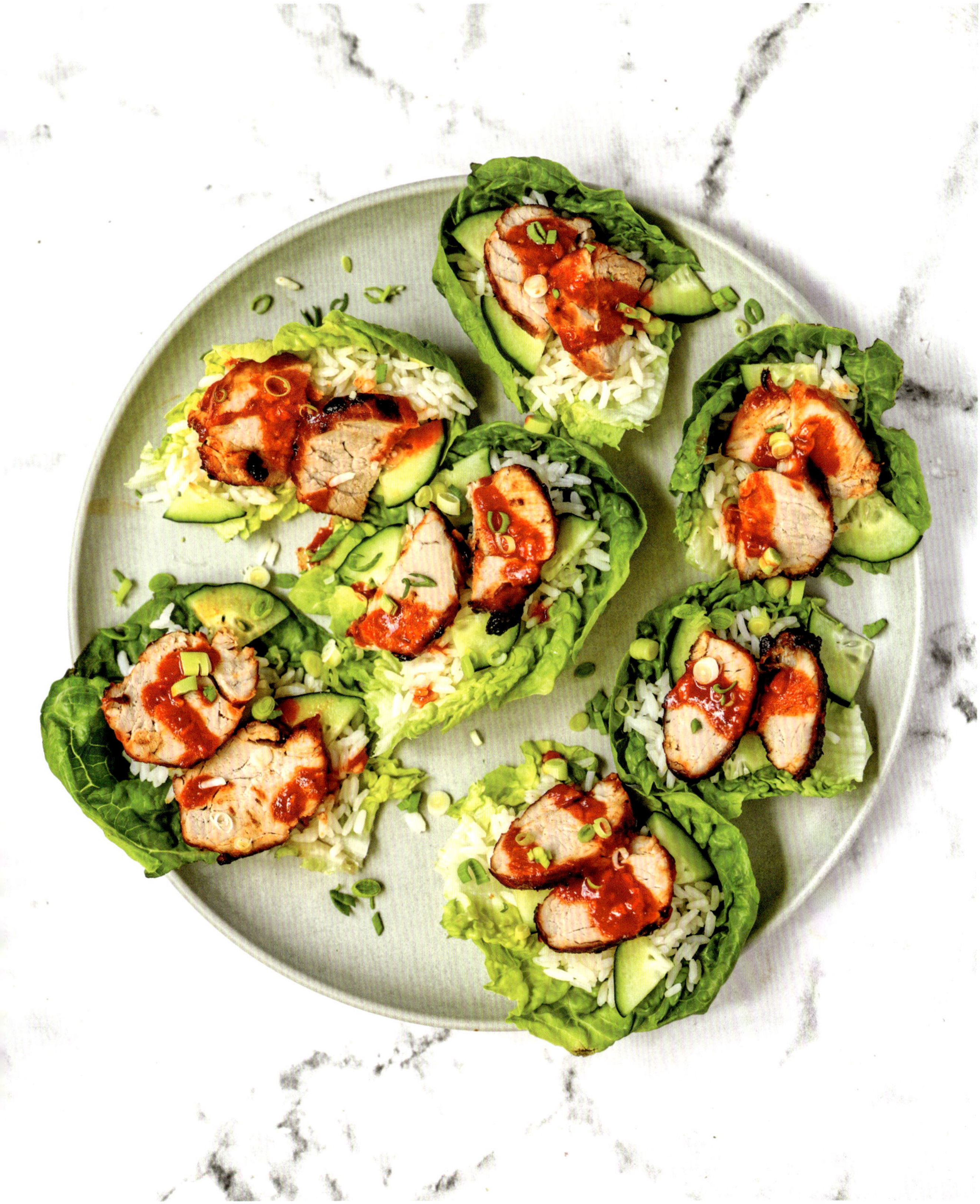

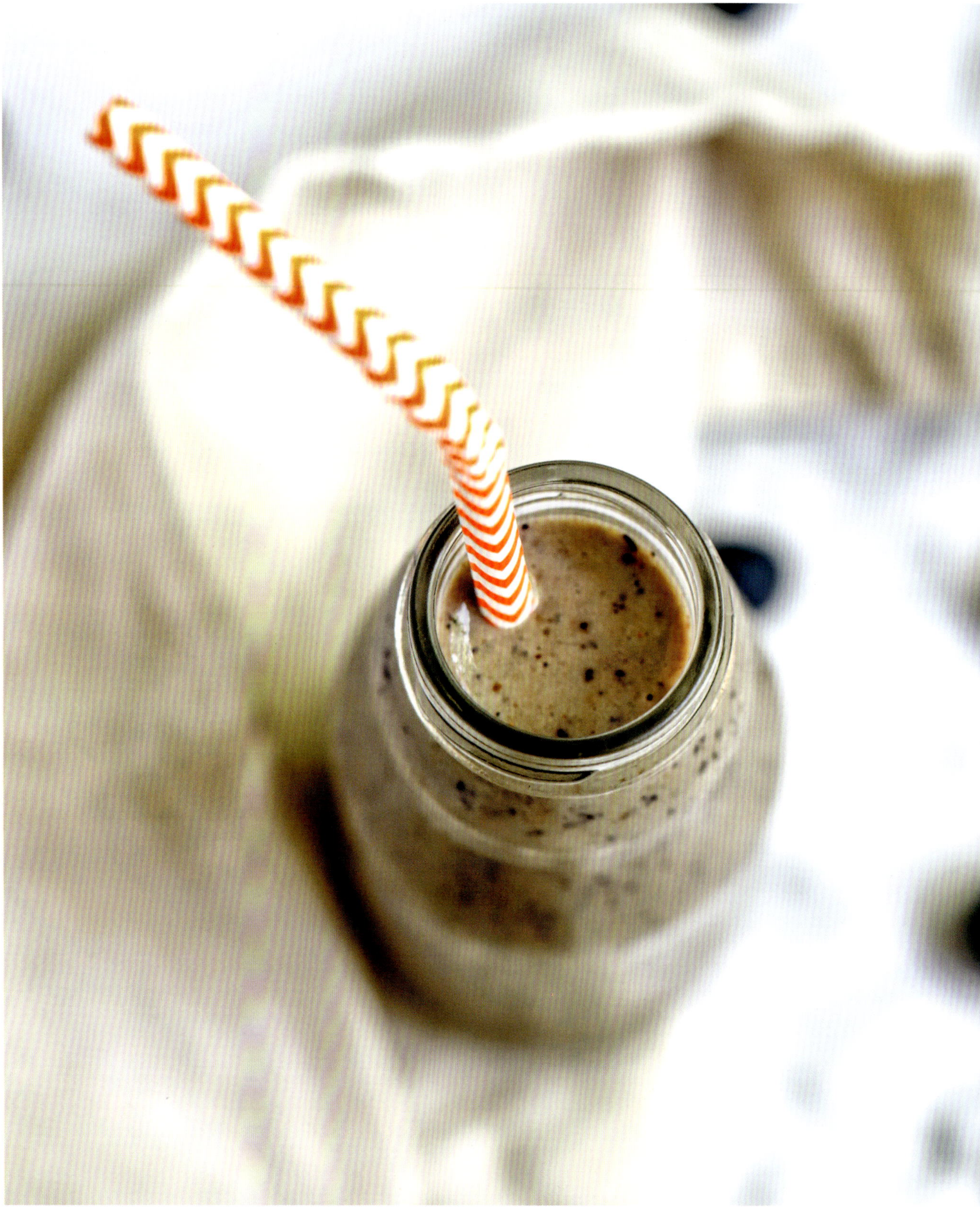

SERVES **1** | **5** MINUTES

BLUEBERRY TAHINI PROTEIN SMOOTHIE

INGREDIENTS

5 fl oz (150 ml) **almond milk**, unsweetened
3.5 oz (100 g) **blueberries**
1 oz (30 g) **vanilla protein powder**
½ **banana**
1 tsp **tahini**
1 tsp **ground cinnamon**
½ tsp **vanilla extract**

METHOD

- Place all the ingredients in a high-speed blender, add a pinch of salt and blend until smooth. Pour into a glass and serve immediately.

ENERGY: **285** Kcal	CARBS: **34** g	PROTEIN: **26** g	FAT: **5** g

MAKES **12** | **20** MINUTES

PROTEIN ALMOND DONUTS

INGREDIENTS

4.8 oz (135 g) **almond meal**
2 oz (60 g) **vanilla protein powder**
1½ tsp **baking powder**
4 fl oz (120 ml) **maple syrup**
2 **large eggs**, at room temperature
4 tbsp **coconut oil**, melted
4 tbsp **unsweetened almond milk**
2 tsp **vanilla extract**
4 tbsp **70% dark chocolate**, melted
1 tbsp **sprinkles**

METHOD

- Preheat the oven to 350°F (180°C). Prepare a 12-hole silicone donut pan.
- Add the almond meal, protein powder, baking powder and 1/4 tsp salt to a bowl and stir until combined. Add the maple syrup, eggs, coconut oil, almond milk and vanilla extract to the same bowl and mix until just combined.
- Divide the batter evenly into each hole in the donut pan. Place into the hot oven and bake for 10 minutes. Remove from the oven and cool in the pan for 2 minutes, then set aside on a wire cooling rack.
- While the donuts are cooling, melt the chocolate. Drizzle the chocolate over the top and sprinkle with some sprinkles.
- Place the donuts into the refrigerator to allow the chocolate to set.
- Storage: place donuts in an airtight container and store at room temperature for 2–3 days or in the refrigerator for 4–5 days.

ENERGY: **213** Kcal | CARBS: **16** g | PROTEIN: **8** g | FAT: **13** g

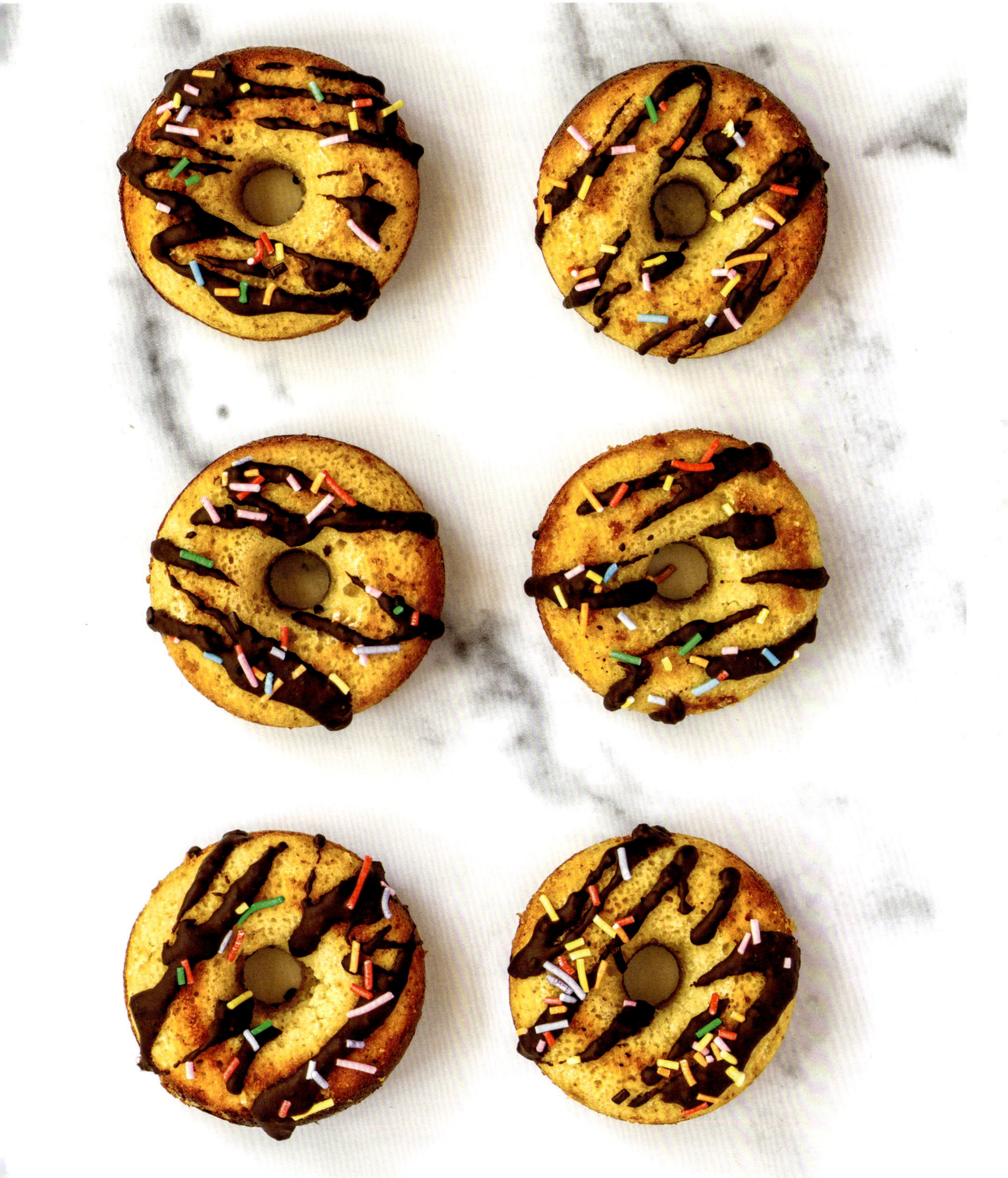

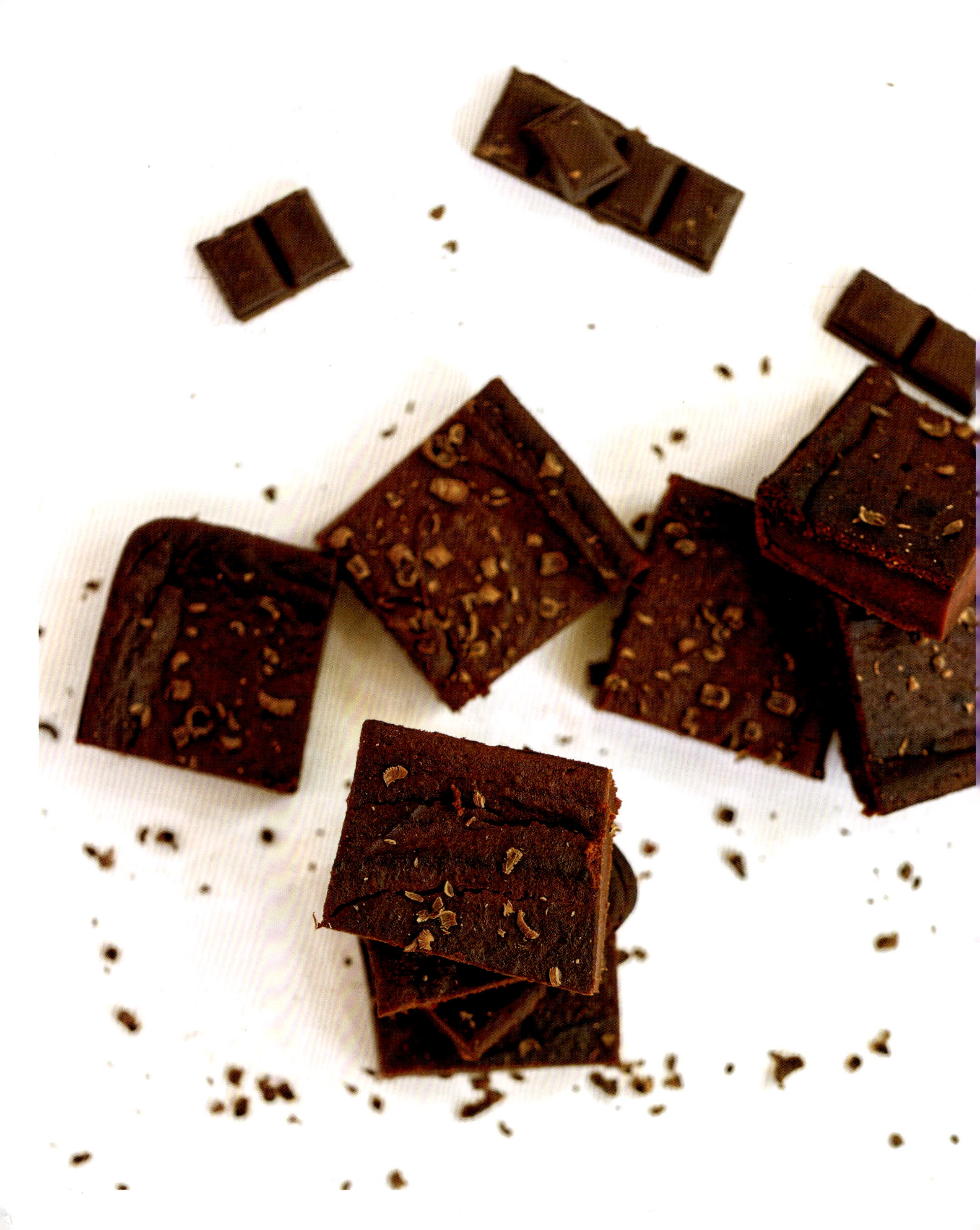

SERVES **9** | **55** MINUTES

BEETROOT CHOCOLATE BROWNIES

INGREDIENTS

3.2 oz (90 g) **70% dark chocolate**
2.7 oz (75 g) **butter**
2.5 oz (70 g) **coconut sugar**
9.9 oz (280 g) **cooked beetroot**, chopped
4.9 oz (140 g) **all-purpose flour**
¼ tsp **baking soda**
½ tsp **baking powder**
2 tsp **unsweetened cocoa powder**
8.8 oz (250 g) **applesauce**

METHOD

- Preheat the oven to 375°F (190°C). Line a 7x9-inch brownie pan with baking paper or use a silicone brownie pan.
- Finely chop the chocolate and melt in a small bowl along with the butter. Once melted, stir in the sugar and set aside.
- Puree the beetroot in a food processor and set aside.
- Add the flour, baking soda, baking powder and cocoa powder to a large mixing bowl and stir well to combine.
- Now add the applesauce, puréed beetroot and melted chocolate. Stir until all ingredients are well combined. Then pour the batter into the prepared pan. Place the pan onto the middle rack of the oven and bake for 40 minutes.
- Remove from the oven and allow the brownies to cool completely in the pan. Once cool, cut into squares and serve.

ENERGY: **231** Kcal	CARBS: **31** g	PROTEIN: **2** g	FAT: **11** g

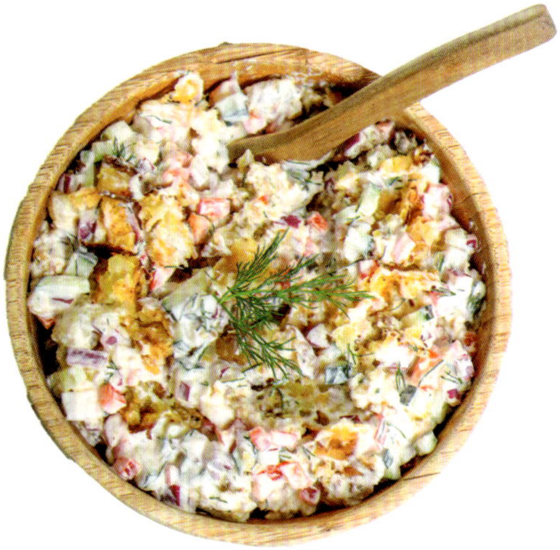

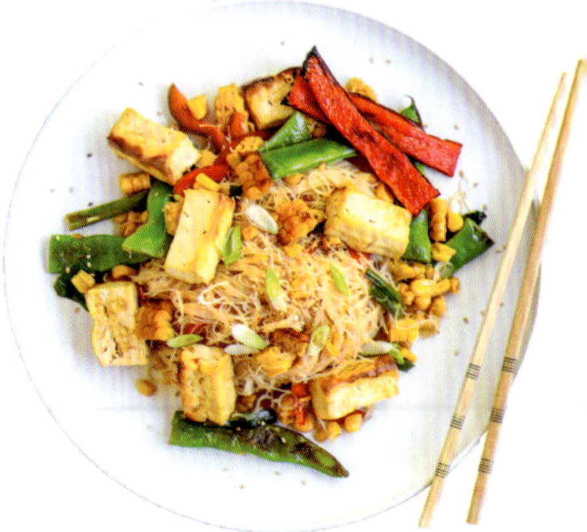

RECIPES WEEK 2

VEGAN CORONATION CHICKPEAS

QUINOA SPINACH TORTILLA

KIWI CHIA PUDDING

ROSEMARY WHITE BEAN DIP

PULLED MUSHROOM WRAPS

SWEET POTATO WRAPS WITH SPICY GUACAMOLE

CRISPY POTATO SALAD

ONE PAN TOFU AND VERMICELLI NOODLE STIR-FRY

ZUCCHINI SOUP

SPICY MAPLE TOFU BOWL

ONE PAN TOMATO AND GNOCCHI BAKE

TURKISH CHICKPEA SALAD

VEGAN TROPICAL SMOOTHIE

CRACKERS

NUT BITES

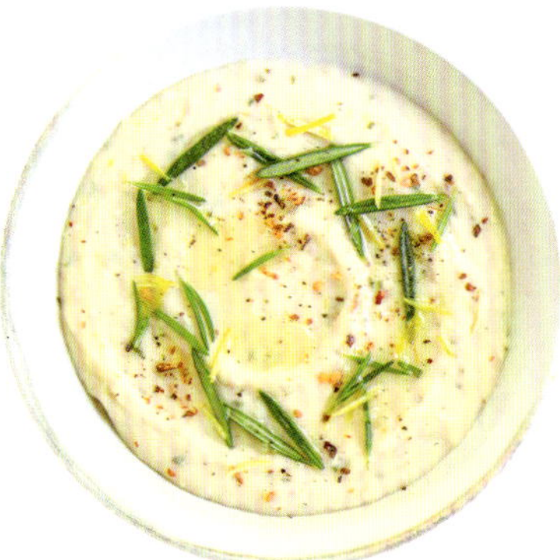

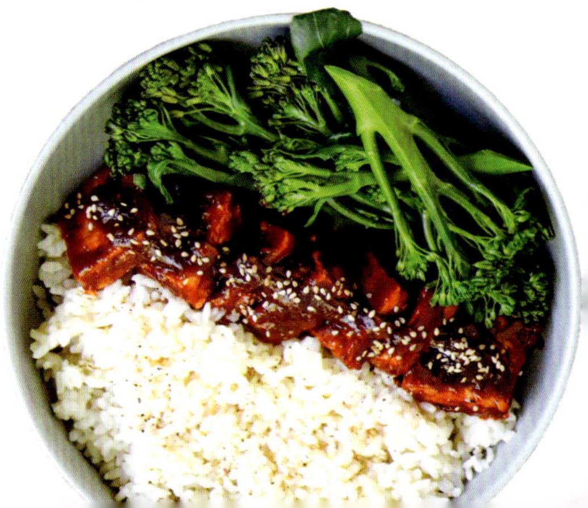

WEEKLY SHOPPING LIST

FRUITS
1 avocado
1 punnet blueberries
4 kiwi fruits
2 lemons
1 lime
1 orange

VEGETABLES
3 onions
2 red onions
bunch green onions
2 bulbs garlic
2 tomatoes
cherry tomatoes
1 cucumber
2 red bell peppers
1 chili pepper
baby spinach
arugula (rocket)
lettuce of choice
green beans
broccolini
red cabbage
2 zucchinis (courgette)
oyster mushrooms
3 carrots
1.7 lb (750 g) potatoes
1 sweet potato

FRESH HERBS
basil
cilantro (coriander)
parsley
rosemary thyme

FROZEN FOODS
pineapple

DRIED
soft dates
raisins

COLD
plant based milk of choice
plant based natural yogurt
vegan feta cheese
1.7 lb (750 g) firm tofu

GRAINS
short grain brown rice

NUTS, SEEDS
coconut flakes
roasted almonds
roasted cashew nuts
roasted peanuts
chia seeds
flaxseeds
quinoa
poppy seeds
pumpkin seeds
sesame seeds
sunflower seeds

BAKING
cornstarch (cornflour)
strong white bread flour (or substitute all-purpose/plain flour)
dark chocolate
vanilla extract

DRIED HERBS, SPICES
black pepper
paprika
smoked paprika
chili powder
red pepper flakes (chili flakes)
garlic powder
ground cumin
ground cloves
ground cinnamon
ground turmeric
sumac
mild curry powder
garam masala

OILS
coconut oil
olive oil
sesame oil
spray cooking oil

SWEETENERS
agave syrup
coconut
sugar
maple syrup

BOXED, CANNED, CONDIMENTS
1 x 7 oz (200 g) can cannellini beans
2 x 14 oz (400 g) cans chickpeas
1 x 2.8 oz (80 g) can corn (sweetcorn)
1 x 3.4 oz (100 g) can coconut milk
2 x 14 oz (400 g) cans cherry tomatoes
1 x 14 oz (400 g) can green lentils
vegan mayonnaise
Dijon mustard
mango chutney
nut butter of choice
sun-dried tomatoes in oil
balsamic vinegar
red wine vinegar
rice wine vinegar
tamari sauce
sriracha sauce
rice
vermicelli noodles
14 oz (400 g) pack gnocchi
sambal oelek or gochujang
vegetable broth (stock)
vegetable stock cubes

MISC/OTHER
sea salt
vegan protein powder

Sample Weekly Meal Planner

	BREAKFAST	LUNCH
Monday	KIWI CHIA PUDDING	SWEET POTATO WRAPS WITH SPICY GUACAMOLE
Tueday	VEGAN CORONATION CHICKPEAS	SWEET POTATO WRAPS WITH SPICY GUACAMOLE
Wednesday	VEGAN CORONATION CHICKPEAS	ZUCCHINI SOUP WITH CRACKERS
Thursday	ROSEMARY WHITE BEAN DIP	PULLED MUSHROOM WRAPS
Friday	ROSEMARY WHITE BEAN DIP	PULLED MUSHROOM WRAPS
Saturday	VEGAN TROPICAL SMOOTHIE	CRISPY POTATO SALAD
Sunday	KIWI CHIA PUDDING	ONE PAN TOMATO AND GNOCCHI BAKE

SNACK	DINNER
E.G. ROSEMARY WHITE BEAN DIP, CRACKERS, NUT BITES, VEGAN TROPICAL SMOOTHIE, KIWI CHIA PUDDING	ONE PAN TOFU AND VERMICELLI NOODLE STIR-FRY
E.G. ROSEMARY WHITE BEAN DIP, CRACKERS, NUT BITES, VEGAN TROPICAL SMOOTHIE, KIWI CHIA PUDDING	ZUCCHINI SOUP WITH CRACKERS
E.G. ROSEMARY WHITE BEAN DIP, CRACKERS, NUT BITES, VEGAN TROPICAL SMOOTHIE, KIWI CHIA PUDDING	SPICY MAPLE TOFU BOWL
E.G. ROSEMARY WHITE BEAN DIP, CRACKERS, NUT BITES, VEGAN TROPICAL SMOOTHIE, KIWI CHIA PUDDING	SPICY MAPLE TOFU BOWL
E.G. ROSEMARY WHITE BEAN DIP, CRACKERS, NUT BITES, VEGAN TROPICAL SMOOTHIE, KIWI CHIA PUDDING	TURKISH CHICKPEA SALAD
E.G. ROSEMARY WHITE BEAN DIP, CRACKERS, NUT BITES, VEGAN TROPICAL SMOOTHIE, KIWI CHIA PUDDING	MEAL OUT – ENJOY!
E.G. ROSEMARY WHITE BEAN DIP, CRACKERS, NUT BITES, VEGAN TROPICAL SMOOTHIE, KIWI CHIA PUDDING	ONE PAN TOFU AND VERMICELLI NOODLE STIR-FRY

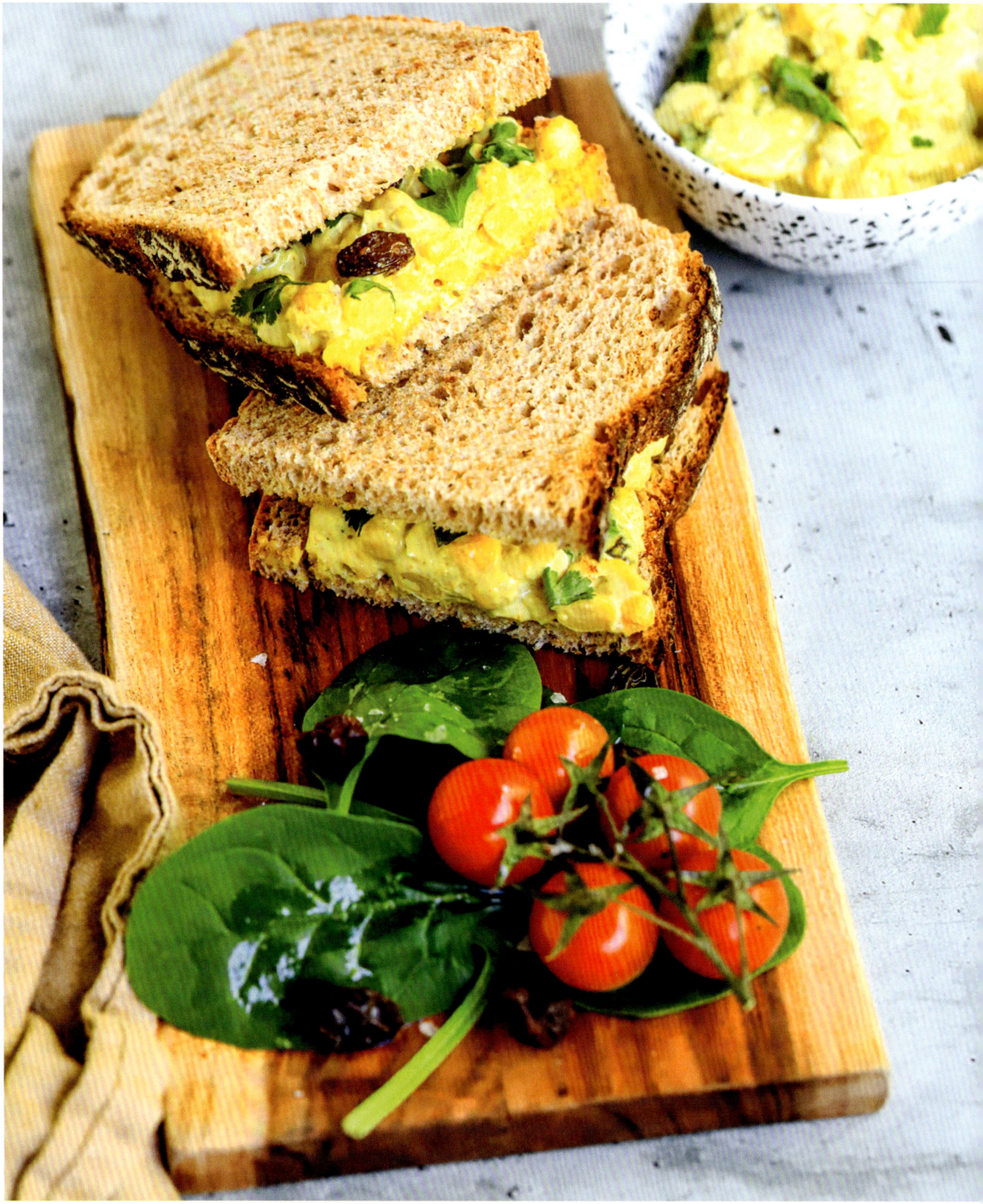

SERVES **4** | **4** MINUTES

VEGAN CORONATION CHICKPEAS

INGREDIENTS

14 oz (400 g) can **chickpeas**, drained
3 tbsp **vegan mayonnaise**
1 tbsp **mango chutney**
1 tsp **mild curry powder**
1 tbsp **raisins**
sea salt and **black pepper** to taste
toasted **bread**, to serve (optional, not included in nutritional breakdown)

METHOD

- Drain and rinse the chickpeas, then place them in a bowl and mash with the back of a fork, or masher, to desired consistency. If you prefer you can leave some whole or don't mash the chickpeas at all.
- Add the vegan mayonnaise, mango chutney, curry powder, raisins, salt and pepper, and stir through.
- This delicious coronation chickpea recipe makes a great sandwich topped with freshly chopped cilantro. Or try topping a jacket potato or add to your favourite salad bowl.

Storage: Store in an airtight container in the refrigerator for up to 3 days.

ENERGY: **197** Kcal | CARBS: **23** g | PROTEIN: **6** g | FAT: **9** g

QUINOA SPINACH **TORTILLA**

INGREDIENTS

7.4 oz (210 g) **quinoa**
3 oz (90 g) **baby spinach**
6 fl oz (180 ml) **water**, at room temperature
½ tsp **salt**
¼ tsp **garlic powder**
spray **cooking oil**, around 1 tbsp

METHOD

- Place the quinoa in a bowl and cover with tap water. Place a plate on top of the bowl and soak it at room temperature for at least 2 hours or overnight.
- Place the soaked quinoa into a sieve and rinse under cold water. Add the drained quinoa into a high-speed blender along with the spinach, water, salt and garlic powder.
- Blend until you achieve a smooth batter. The batter should not be thick, and no pieces of quinoa should be left whole at the end. Transfer the batter into a mixing bowl.
- Warm a non-stick skillet over medium heat and spray with cooking oil. Pour ½ cup of the batter into the centre of the skillet, and using the back of a spoon, work in a circular motion to gently spread the batter from the centre to the outside edge until it forms a 5" (12 cm) tortilla.
- Cook for 2 minutes on one side, then use a rubber spatula to flip over, and cook for 1 minute on the second side.
- Set the cooked tortillas down on a wire rack to cool. Don't stack them warm without adding a piece of parchment paper between them, or they will stick together.
- Storage: Store in the fridge in a sealed box for up to 3 days, making sure the quinoa tortillas don't touch and overlap, as they can stick together. Reheat the tortillas in a warm, non-stick pan or sandwich press if wrapped with filling.

ENERGY: **148** Kcal	CARBS: **23** g	PROTEIN: **5** g	FAT: **4** g

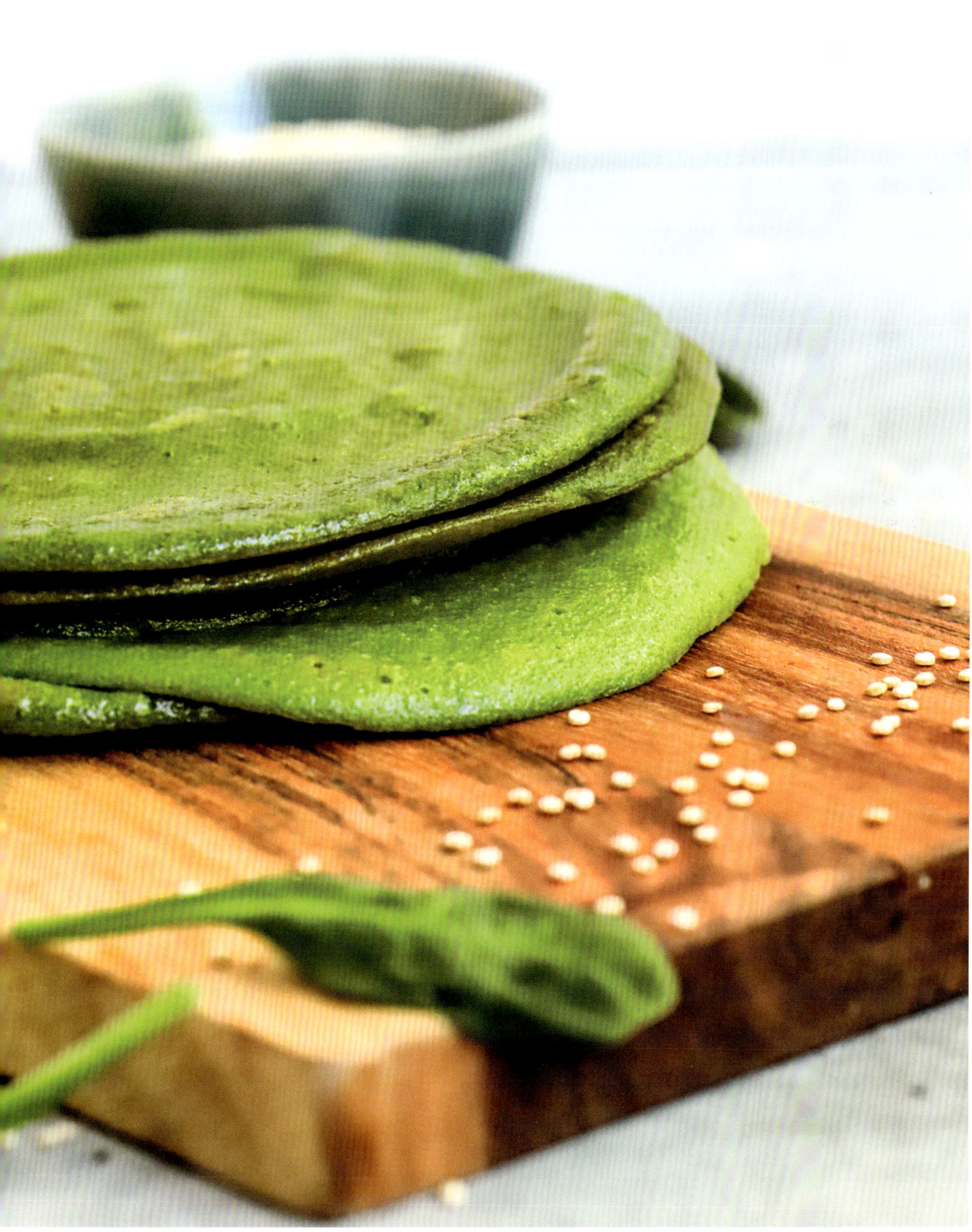

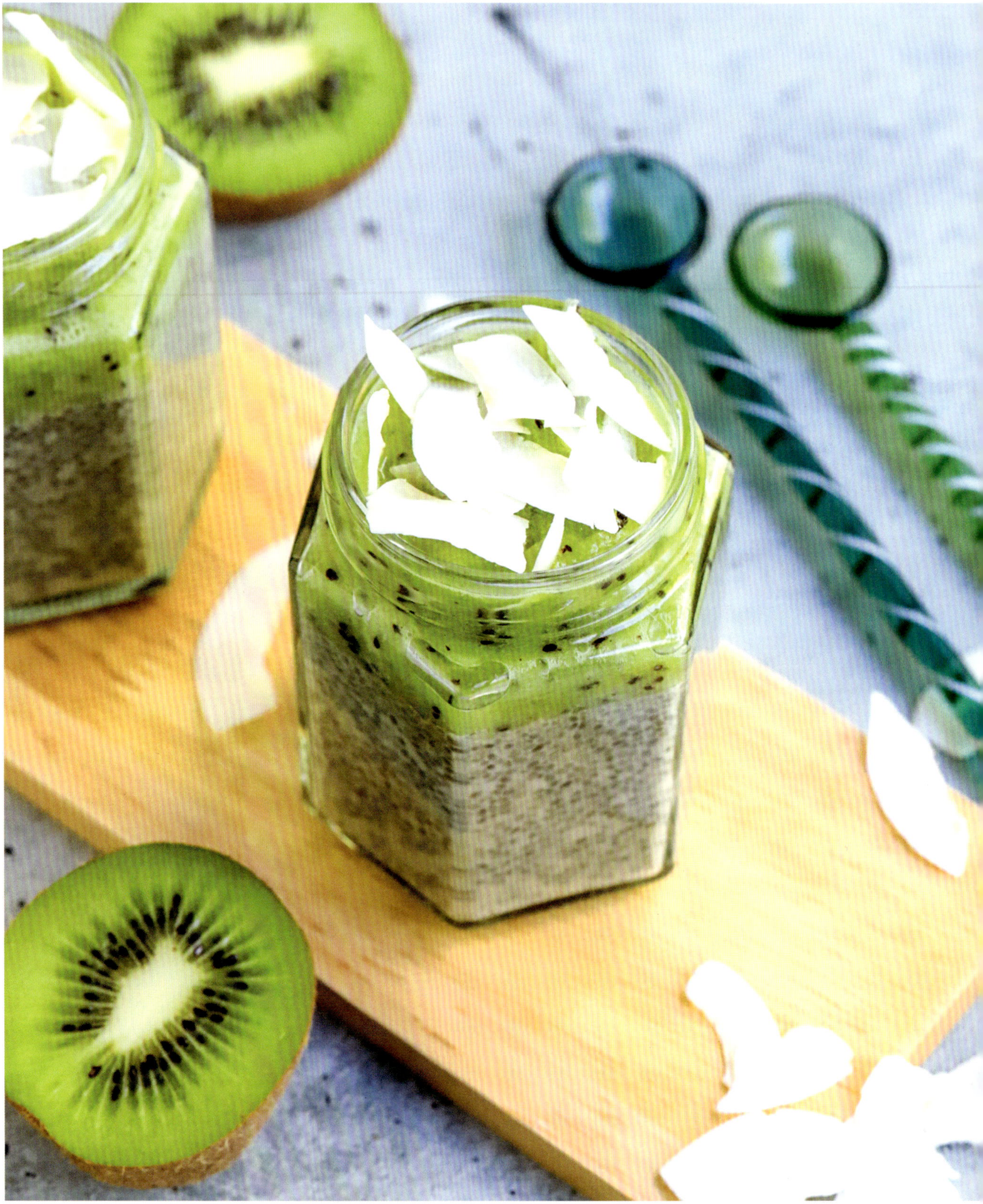

KIWI CHIA PUDDING

INGREDIENTS

4.9 oz (140 g) **chia seeds**
12 fl oz (360 ml) **plant-based milk** of choice
1¼ tbsp **agave syrup**
1 tsp **vanilla extract**
4 **kiwi**, peeled
3.5 oz (100 g) **fresh blueberries**
1 tbsp **toasted coconut flakes**

METHOD

- Place the chia seeds, milk, agave syrup and vanilla extract in a bowl, and stir well to combine.
- Divide the mixture between 3 small serving jars, cover, and place in the refrigerator for at least 1–2 hours.
- Give the puddings a quick stir from time to time to ensure that the seeds absorb most of the liquid.
- Meanwhile, place 3 kiwis into a blender and blitz to a smooth purée. Chop the remaining kiwi into small pieces.
- Assemble the kiwi chia pudding by topping the creamy base with the kiwi purée, chopped kiwi, blueberries and toasted coconut flakes.
- Storage: Cover and store the chia pudding in the refrigerator for up to 5 days.

ENERGY: **369** kcal | CARBS: **44** g | PROTEIN: **10** g | FAT: **17** g

SERVES **2** | **15** MINUTES

ROSEMARY WHITE BEAN **DIP**

INGREDIENTS

2 tbsp **olive oil**
1 clove **garlic**, minced
2 sprigs **rosemary**, remove needles, chop
7 oz (200 g) **cannellini beans**, drained and rinsed
½ **lemon**, zest and juice
sea salt and **black pepper**
½ **red pepper** flakes

METHOD

- Heat the olive oil over medium heat and sauté the garlic and rosemary. Add the beans and lemon zest, warm through.
- Add the contents of the pot to a food processor and purée until the dip reaches the desired consistency.
- Season to taste with lemon juice, salt, pepper and chili flakes.
- Serve the dip with vegetable sticks or bread (not included in nutritional breakdown).

ENERGY: **218** Kcal	CARBS: **19** g	PROTEIN: **4** g	FAT: **14** g

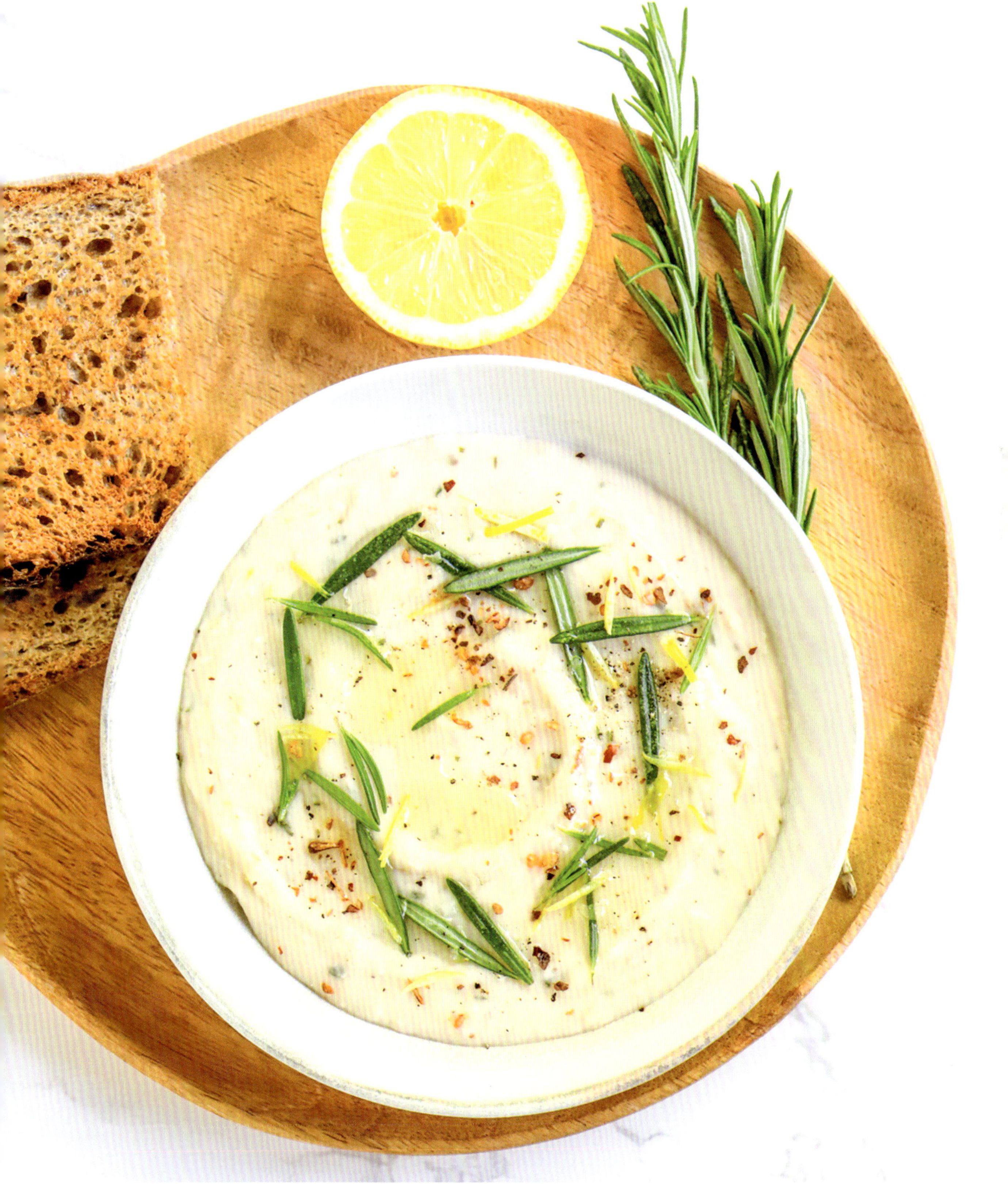

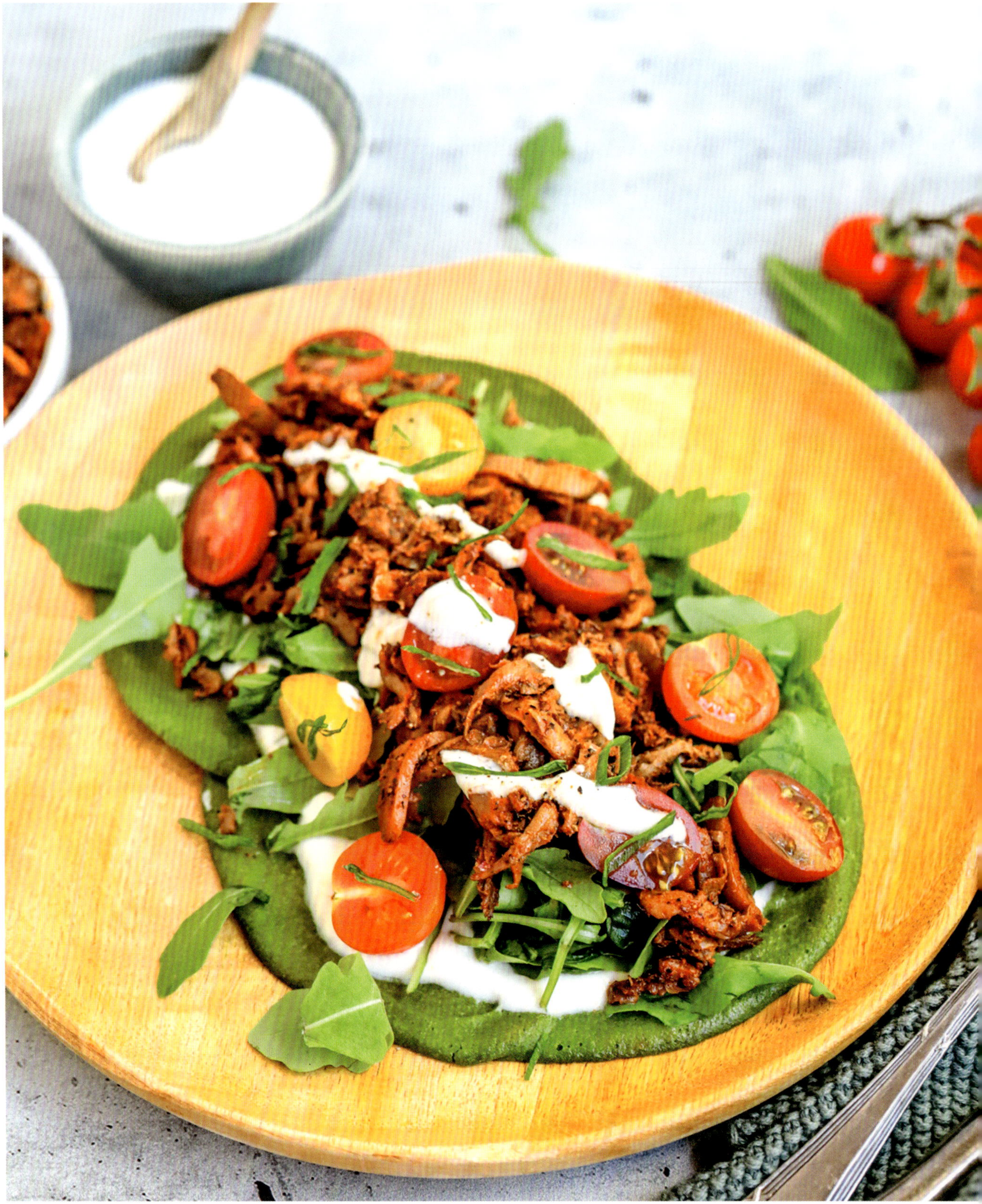

PULLED MUSHROOM WRAPS

INGREDIENTS

10.6 oz (300 g) **oyster mushrooms**
4 tbsp **olive oil**
2 tsp **paprika**
1 tsp **thyme**
sea salt and **black pepper**, to taste
2 **quinoa spinach tortillas** (see recipe on page 60)
3.5 oz (100 g) **plant-based natural yogurt**
1.4 oz (40 g) **arugula**
7 oz (200 g) **cherry tomatoes**, quartered
2 tsp **balsamic vinegar**
4 tbsp **parsley**, chopped

METHOD

- Using a fork, shred the stems of the mushrooms and slice the caps into pieces.
- Heat the olive oil in a skillet and add the mushrooms, paprika and thyme. Mix well and sauté for 6 minutes, then season to taste with salt and pepper. Remove the mushrooms from the skillet, set aside, and heat the tortillas.
- Spread some of the Greek yogurt on each tortilla. Top with the mushrooms, arugula and tomatoes, then season with balsamic vinegar, salt and pepper.
- Drizzle the wraps with the remaining yogurt, garnish with parsley and serve.

ENERGY: 505 Kcal | CARBS: 40 g | PROTEIN: 12 g | FAT: 33 g

SERVES **2** | **20** MINUTES

SWEET POTATO WRAPS WITH SPICY GUACAMOLE

INGREDIENTS

1 **sweet potato**, peeled
2 **carrots**, peeled
2 tbsp **olive oil**
sea salt and **black pepper**, to taste
½ **avocado**
2 **tomatoes**, chopped
1 **red onion**, half diced, half sliced
½ **chili pepper**, deseeded and diced
4 tbsp **cilantro**, chopped
½ **lime**, juiced
2 **quinoa spinach tortillas** (see recipe on page 60)
handful of **lettuce**
2 oz (60 g) **vegan feta**

METHOD

- Preheat the oven to 400°F (200°C). Line a baking sheet with baking paper.
- Cut the sweet potatoes and carrots into batons and place on the lined baking sheet. Drizzle with olive oil and season with salt and pepper. Place in the hot oven to bake for about 20 minutes.
- Place the avocado flesh in a bowl and mash with a fork. Mix in the diced onion, chili and cilantro. Add the lime juice and season to taste with salt and pepper.
- To serve, heat the tortillas, then spread with the guacamole. Top each tortilla with the baked sweet potato and carrot, then add the lettuce, tomato, sliced onion and crumbled feta.

ENERGY: **594** Kcal | CARBS: **62** g | PROTEIN: **10** g | FAT: **34** g

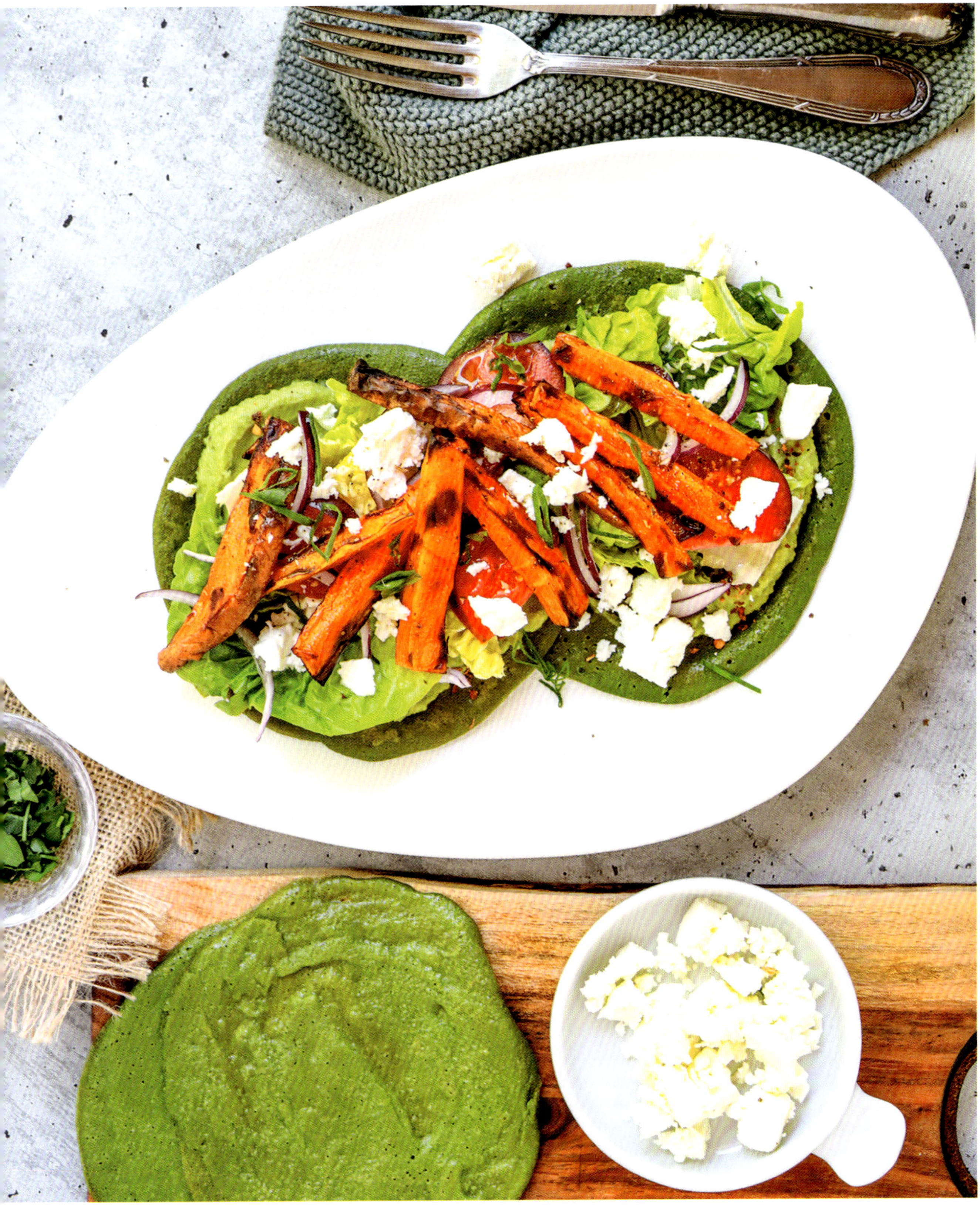

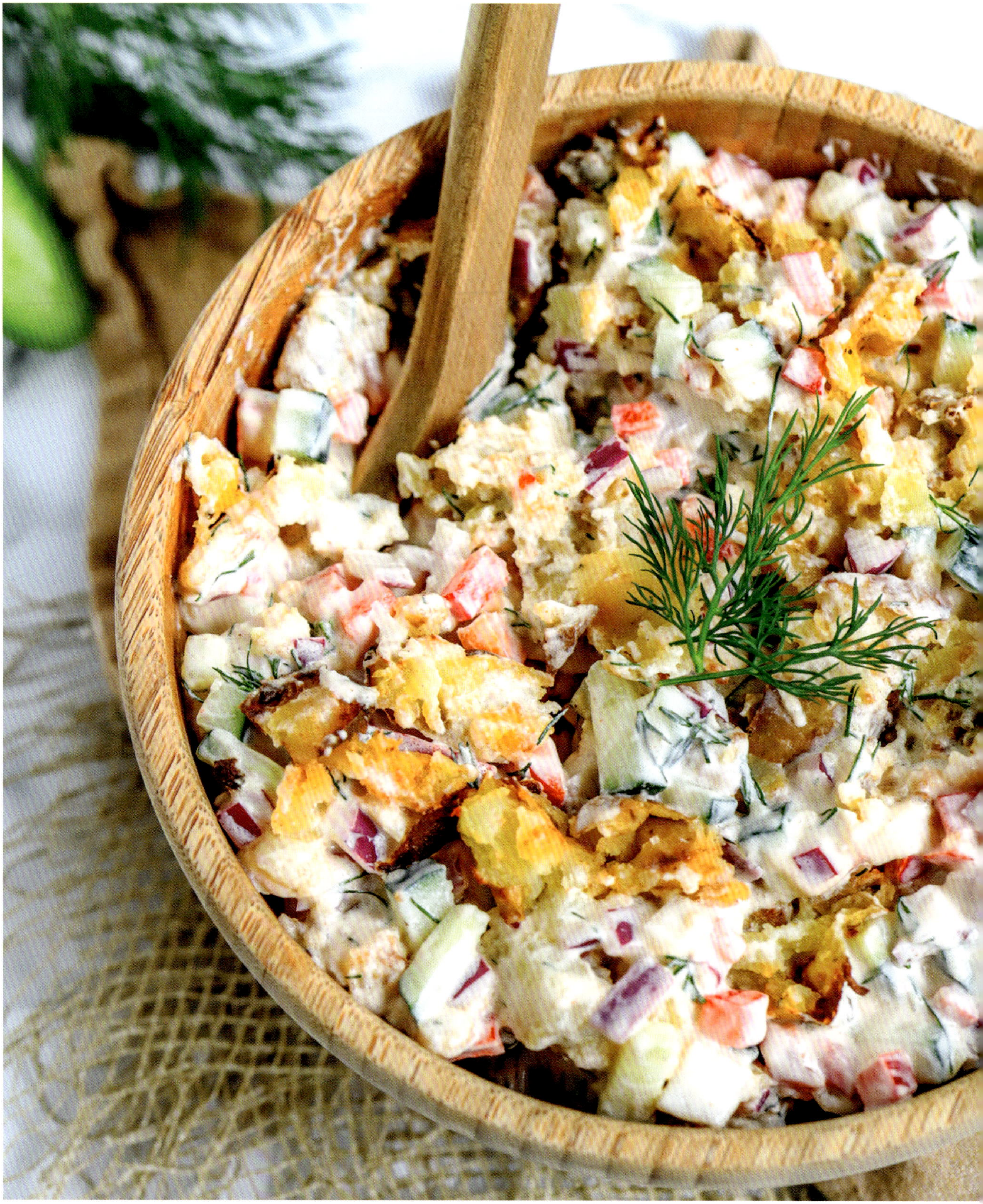

SERVES **4** | **20** MINUTES

CRISPY POTATO SALAD

INGREDIENTS

1.3 lb (600 g) **potatoes**
1 tbsp **olive oil**
sea salt and **black pepper**, to taste
½ **cucumber**, chopped
½ **red bell pepper**, chopped
1 **red onion**, diced
2 tbsp **dill**, chopped

For the dressing

4 tbsp **plant based natural yogurt**
2 tbsp **vegan mayonnaise**
1 tbsp **mustard**
½ **lemon**, juiced
sea salt and **black pepper**

METHOD

- Preheat the oven to 350°F (180°C).
- Boil the potatoes, then drain them and place on a tray and mash them. Add some olive oil and season with salt and pepper. Bake in the oven for about 20 minutes.
- Place all the ingredients for the dressing into a large bowl and mix well to combine. Add the remaining salad vegetables, along with the baked potatoes and serve immediately.

ENERGY: **217** Kcal	CARBS: **30** g	PROTEIN: **4** g	FAT: **9** g

SERVES **2** | **10** MINUTES

ONE PAN TOFU AND VERMICELLI NOODLE STIR-FRY

INGREDIENTS

For the stir-fry sauce

3 tbsp **tamari**

1½ tbsp **rice wine vinegar**

2 tsp **maple syrup**

1 tsp **toasted sesame oil**

1 **garlic clove**, finely grated

1–2 tsp **sriracha sauce**

For the noodles

1 tsp **coconut oil**

5.3 oz (150) **green beans**

½ **red bell pepper**, sliced

2.8 oz (80 g) **corn**, drained

3 **green onions**, sliced, keep green tops to garnish

12 fl oz (360 ml) **water**

3.5 oz (100 g) **rice vermicelli noodles**

2 oz (60 g) **roasted peanuts**

For the tofu

10.6 oz (300 g) **firm tofu**, pressed

1½ tbsp **tamari sauce**

1 tbsp **water**

1 tsp **coconut oil**, melted

METHOD

- To make the stir fry sauce, place all the sauce ingredients into a jar, screw the lid on tight, and shake well to emulsify. (Leftover sauce can be stored in the refrigerator for 1–2 weeks.)
- To make the noodles, start by preheating a wok until hot. Add a teaspoon of coconut oil, swirl it around the wok and add the green beans. Stir-fry for 1–2 minutes then add the bell pepper, corn and spring onion segments. Add another teaspoon of oil. Carry on stir-frying until all the veggies are no longer raw and charred in places.
- Remove the veggies from the wok and set aside. Pour the water into the wok and place the noodles on top. After a few seconds, flip the noodles using kitchen tongs. Cook the noodles until all of the liquid has been absorbed, then carry on cooking them for a little longer.
- Stir the sauce through the softened noodles, add the vegetables back into the wok, along with the optional tofu (see instructions below) if using. Stir-fry everything for a few seconds to warm through, then divide equally between 2 bowls, top with peanuts and additional spring onion tops, and serve.

TOFU – OPTIONAL

- Preheat the oven to 400°F (200°C). Line a large baking sheet with baking paper.
- Cut the firm tofu into ½" (1.25 cm) cubes. Combine the tamari sauce and water in a large, flat bottomed dish and coat the cubes of tofu in the liquid. Set aside to marinate for at least 1 hour, stirring occasionally.
- Lift the tofu out of the marinade and arrange it on the lined baking sheet. Place in the hot oven to bake for 15 minutes.
- Stir the coconut oil through the tofu and return to the oven for a further 15 minutes (if using a pressed brand of tofu, like Tofu, 5–10 minutes is enough).

ENERGY: **687** Kcal | CARBS: **73** g | PROTEIN: **29** g | FAT: **31** g

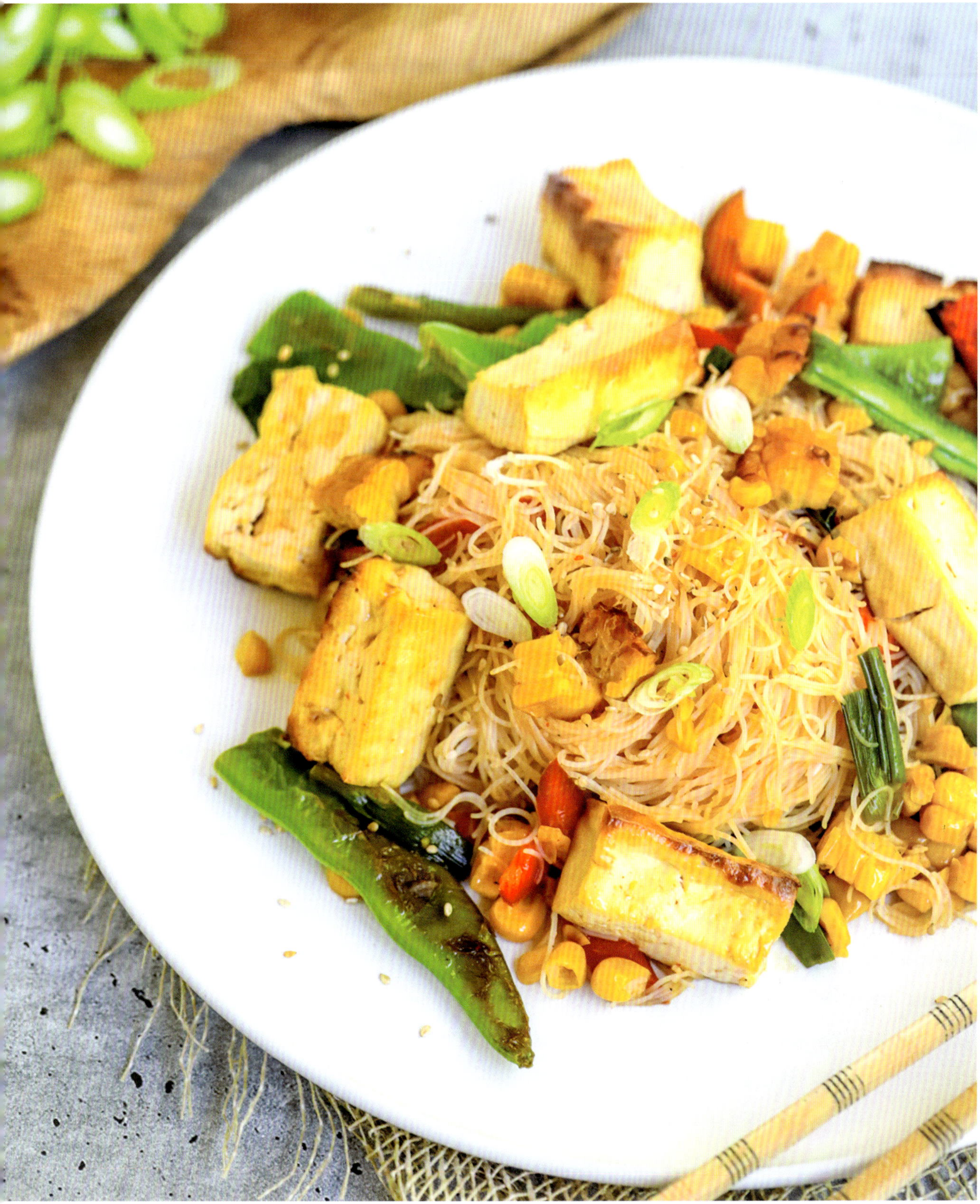

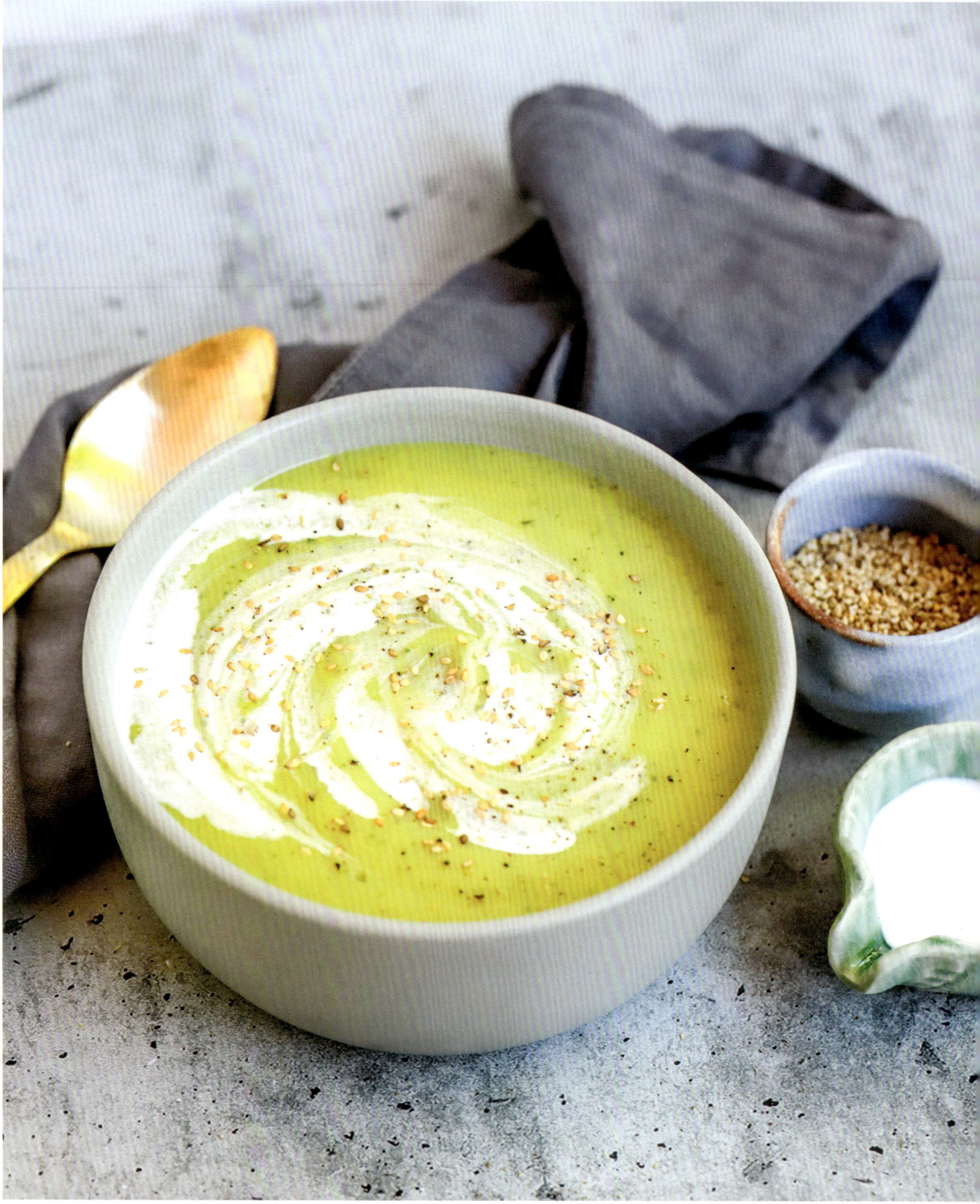

SERVES **2** | **20** MINUTES

ZUCCHINI SOUP

INGREDIENTS

1 tbsp **olive oil**
1 **onion**, diced
1 **clove garlic**, minced
5.3 oz (150 g) **potatoes**, peeled and diced
2 **zucchinis**, diced
1 **carrot**, peeled and chopped
1.5 pints (700 ml) **vegetable broth**
sea salt and **black pepper**, to taste
0.4 oz (10 g) **sesame seeds**
3.4 fl oz (100 ml) can **coconut milk, light**

METHOD

- Heat the olive oil in a large pot over medium heat and sauté the onions and garlic for 3 minutes. Add the potatoes and cook for a further 4 minutes, then add the zucchini, carrot and vegetable broth and bring to a boil. Season with salt and pepper, reduce the heat and simmer for 15 minutes.
- In the meantime, lightly toast the sesame seeds in a dry non-stick skillet, taking care not to burn the seeds.
- Once soup has finished cooking, purée with an immersion blender and add the coconut milk.
- Pour the soup into 2 small bowls, sprinkle with the toasted sesame seeds and serve. Serve with bean dip and crackers.

ENERGY: **273** Kcal | CARBS: **33** g | PROTEIN: **6** g | FAT: **13** g

SPICY MAPLE TOFU BOWL

INGREDIENTS

For the garlic rice

2 tsp **olive oil**
1 clove **garlic**, finely grated with a microplane
½ tsp **ground turmeric**
7.4 oz (210 g) **short grain brown rice**, rinsed well and drained
14 fl oz (420 ml) **vegetable broth**
sea salt and **black pepper**, to taste

For the tofu and broccolini

1 lb (450 g) **firm tofu**, drained, cubed
1 tbsp **cornstarch**
sea salt and **black pepper**, to taste
2 fl oz (60 g) **maple syrup**
2 tbsp **sambal oelek** or **gochujang**
2 tbsp **tamari sauce**
3 tbsp **rice vinegar**
1 clove **garlic**, minced
7 oz (200 g) **broccolini water**
2 fl oz (60 ml) **olive oil**
sliced **green onions**, for garnish

METHOD

- To make the rice, place a medium pot over medium heat. Add the olive oil and swirl it around, then add the garlic and turmeric and sauté until fragrant, about 30 seconds.
- Add the rice to the pot and stir to coat in the oily spice mixture. Add the vegetable broth, salt, and pepper, and bring to a boil. Once boiling, lower the heat to a simmer, place a lid on top, and cook until all liquid has been absorbed and rice grains are tender, about 45 minutes. Take the rice off the heat.
- Meanwhile, place the tofu cubes on a clean kitchen towel and press to remove any excess moisture. Place the tofu in a bowl and toss with the cornstarch, salt and pepper, then set aside.
- In a small bowl, whisk together the maple syrup, sambal oelek, tamari, rice vinegar and garlic. Set aside.
- Trim the ends off the broccolini and cut any thick stalks in half lengthwise. Set a medium nonstick skillet over medium heat. Pour enough water into the skillet to cover the base of the pan. Bring to a simmer, add the broccolini, and put the lid on top. Steam the broccolini for around 5 minutes, until bright green but still firm. Remove the broccolini, set aside on a plate and season with salt and pepper.
- Wipe out the skillet and return it to the stove over medium heat. Pour in the olive oil, and once the oil is hot, carefully add half of the tofu to the skillet. Let the tofu pieces sit

ENERGY: **419** Kcal | CARBS: **62** g | PROTEIN: **18** g | FAT: **11** g

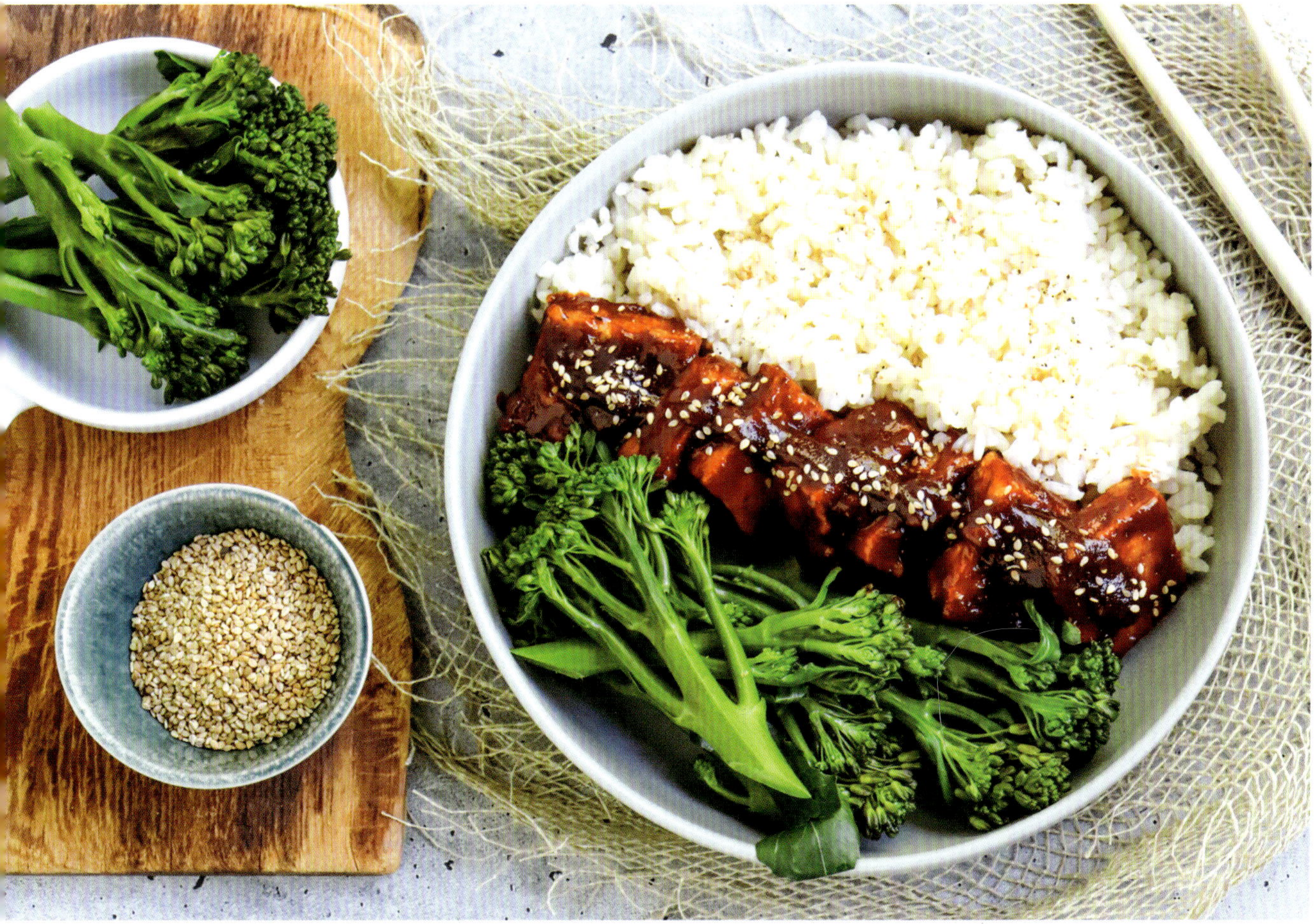

until deeply browned on the bottom, about 3–5 minutes. Carefully flip the pieces over and brown the other side as deeply as you can, this should take a further 3–5 minutes. Place the tofu on a plate and repeat this cooking process with the remaining tofu, adding more oil if necessary.

- Get all the tofu back into the skillet and pour over the maple syrup and sambal oelek mixture. Bring the liquid to a boil, then turn down the heat and simmer until slightly thickened, spooning the sauce over the tofu as the sauce reduces. Once the liquid has reduced by half, around 5 minutes, add the broccolini to the skillet and toss in the warm sauce.
- Serve the spicy maple tofu and broccolini with the golden garlic rice and sliced green onions.

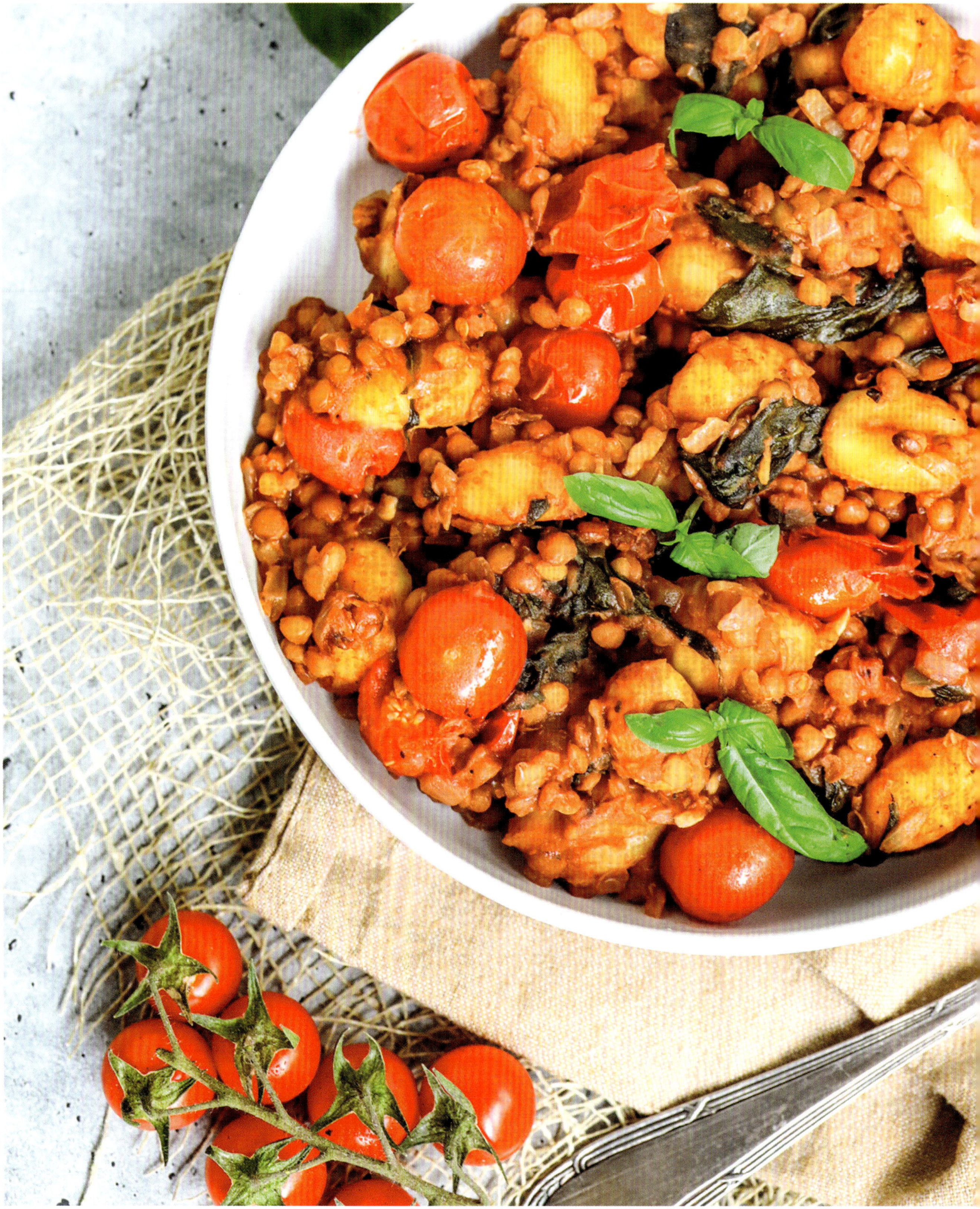

ONE PAN TOMATO AND GNOCCHI **BAKE**

INGREDIENTS

1 tbsp **olive oil**, plus extra to drizzle
1 **onion**, finely chopped
3 cloves **garlic**, grated
14 oz (400 g) **cherry tomatoes**
5 fl oz (150 ml) **hot water**
1 tbsp **balsamic vinegar**
1 tbsp **maple syrup**
1 **vegetable stock cube**, chopped
5–6 **fresh basil leaves**, chopped
2 tbsp **fresh lemon juice**
½ small bunch of **basil**, plus extra to garnish
7 oz (200 g) **spinach**, roughly chopped
1 x 14 oz (400 g) can **green lentils**, drained and rinsed
14 oz (400 g) pack **gnocchi**
pinch of **sea salt** and **black pepper**
pinch of **red pepper** flakes, optional garnish

METHOD

- Preheat the oven to 400°F (200°C).
- To make the tomato sauce, place the olive oil in a shallow oven safe casserole on the stove, over medium heat. Add the onion and fry for 8 minutes until softened, then add the garlic and fry for 30 seconds until fragrant.
- Add the tomatoes, hot water, balsamic vinegar, maple syrup, crumble in the stock cube and stir. Bring to the boil and then stir through the basil and spinach, cooking until wilted.
- Mix in the lentils and gnocchi and stir to combine. Drizzle over some more olive oil, season with sea salt and black pepper and bake in the hot oven for 25 minutes.
- Serve the bake, garnish with a pinch of red pepper flakes (optional) and some basil leaves.

ENERGY: **329** Kcal	CARBS: **58** g	PROTEIN: **13** g	FAT: **5** g

TURKISH CHICKPEA SALAD

INGREDIENTS

For the chickpeas

4 tbsp **olive oil**, divided
14 oz (400 g) can **chickpeas**, drained and rinsed
1 tsp **garam masala**
1 tsp **smoked paprika**
½ tsp **ground cinnamon**
½ tsp **sea salt**
¼ tsp **ground turmeric**
¼ tsp **ground cloves**
¼ tsp **black pepper**, or to taste

For the vegetables

1 **onion**, thinly sliced
4 cloves **garlic**, minced
1 **red pepper**, thinly sliced
2 tbsp **sun dried tomatoes in oil**, finely chopped
½ tsp **sea salt**
1 tbsp **red wine vinegar**
1 tbsp **sumac**
½ tsp **chili powder**
½ tsp **ground cumin**
½ tsp **coconut sugar**, optional
3.5 oz (100 g) **red cabbage**, chopped
0.7 oz (20 g) **cilantro**

METHOD

- To make the chickpeas, place a large skillet over medium heat. Add 2 tablespoons of olive oil and chickpeas to the skillet and stir the chickpeas for 1 minute to coat them in the oil. Now add all the remaining chickpea spices and cook for 5 minutes until the chickpeas are red and fragrant. Pour the chickpeas into a large bowl, scraping in all the spices from the skillet.
- In the same skillet, over medium heat, add the remaining 2 tablespoons of olive oil, then add the onions and garlic. Stir frequently and cook for 3–4 minutes until the onions are slightly soft and the garlic is fragrant. Add the red peppers, sun dried tomatoes and salt, stir and cook for 2 minutes.
- Remove from the heat and set aside to cool slightly. Then add the red wine vinegar and remaining spices, stirring well to combine.
- Add the vegetables to the bowl with the chickpeas, along with the red cabbage, cilantro, basil and lemon juice. Mix together until well combined.
- Serve the salad warm or cold.

ENERGY: 276 Kcal	CARBS: 26 g	PROTEIN: 7 g	FAT: 16 g

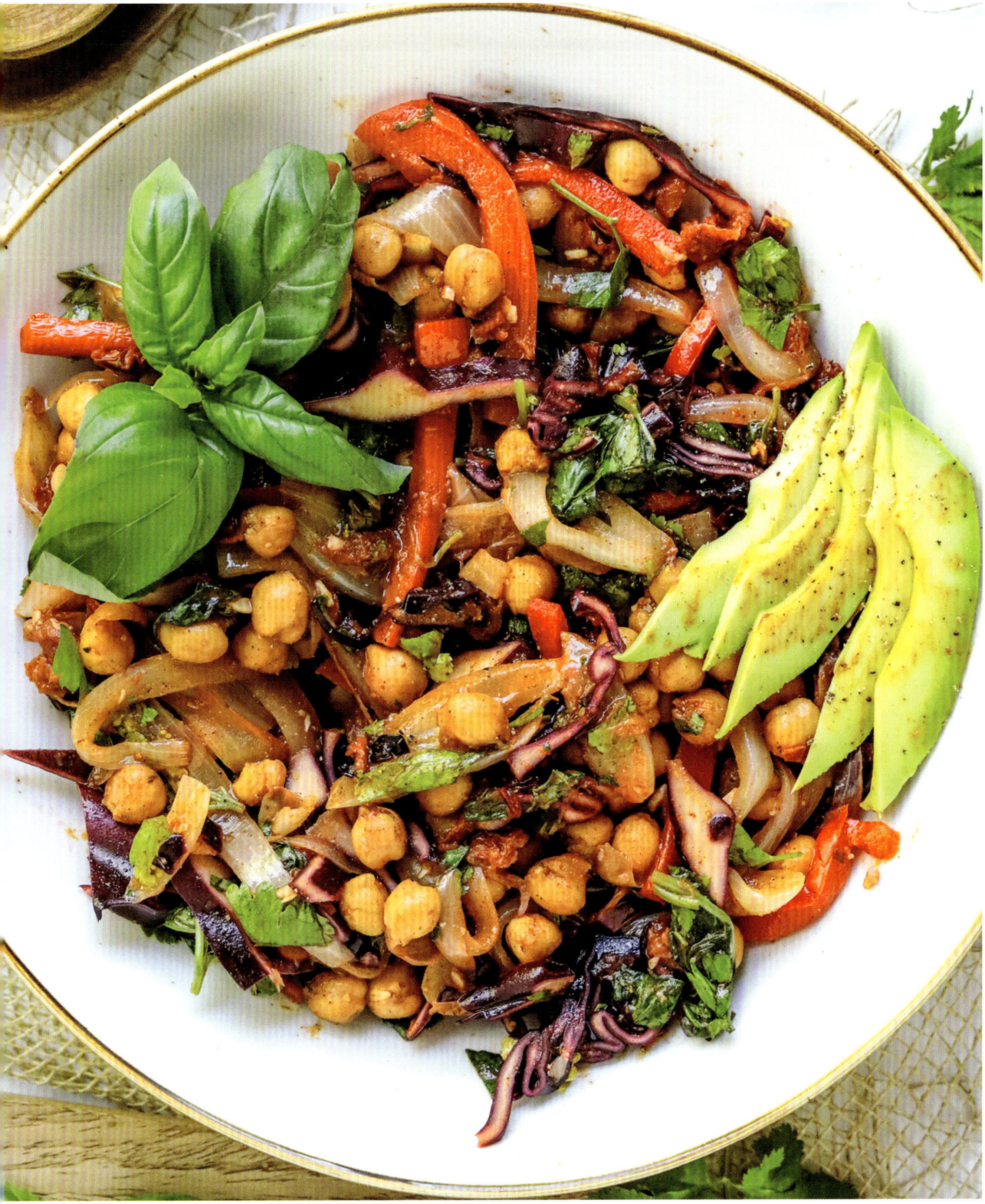

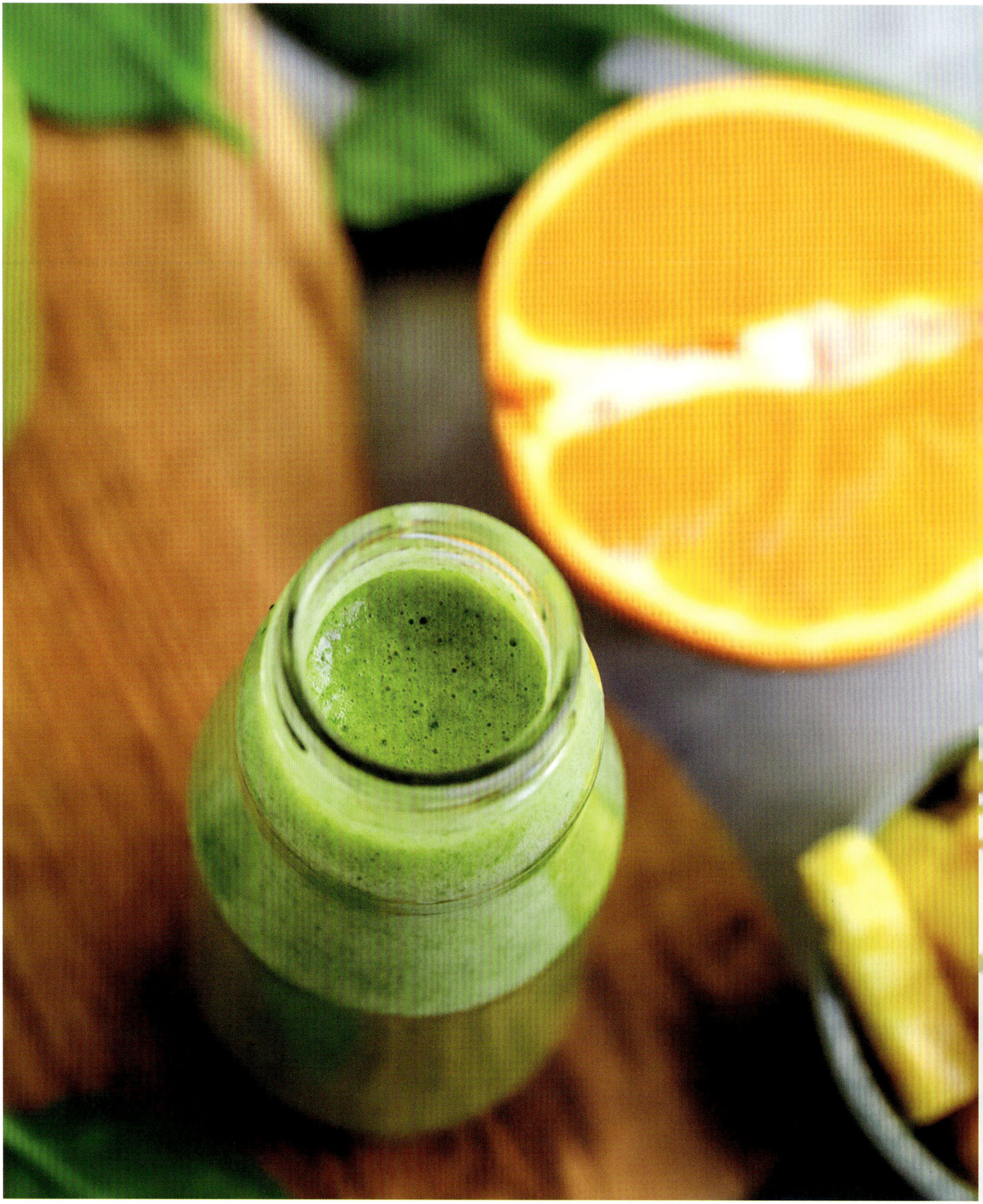

SERVES **1** | **5** MINUTES

VEGAN TROPICAL **SMOOTHIE**

INGREDIENTS

1 oz (30 g) **spinach**
½ **orange**, peeled
4 fl oz (120 ml) **water**
3.9 oz (110 g) **frozen pineapple**
½ **banana**
1 oz (30 g) **vegan protein powder**, optional

METHOD

- Place the spinach, orange and water into a high speed blender and blend until smooth.
- Now add the remaining ingredients into the blender, and blend again until smooth.
- Pour the smoothie into a glass and serve.

ENERGY: **273** Kcal	CARBS: **48** g	PROTEIN: **18** g	FAT: **1** g

MAKES **64** CRACKERS | **45** MINUTES

CRACKERS

INGREDIENTS

8.8 oz (250 g) **all-purpose flour**
0.9 oz (25 g) **pumpkin seeds**
0.9 oz (25 g) **flaxseed**
0.9 oz (25 g) **sunflower seeds**
0.5 oz (15 g) **sesame seeds**
0.2 oz (5 g) **poppy seeds**
4 tbsp **olive oil**
0.2 oz (5 g) **fine sea salt**
3.9 fl oz (100 g) **water**

METHOD

- Preheat the oven to 335°F (170°C). Line 2 baking sheets with baking paper.
- Weigh all the ingredients into a mixing bowl of a stand mixer and combine for 15 seconds at speed 3.
- Knead the dough for 1–2 minutes then tip out onto a lightly floured work surface. Halve the dough and roll out each portion very thinly (1–2 mm thick).
- Cut the dough into squares or rectangles or use a cookie cutter. Place the crackers onto the prepared baking sheet.
- Place the baking sheet into the hot oven and bake for 20–25 minutes. Remove the crackers from the oven and place on a wire rack to cool completely.
- Once cool, store the crackers in an airtight container on the countertop.

ENERGY: **34** Kcal	CARBS: **3** g	PROTEIN: **1** g	FAT: **2** g

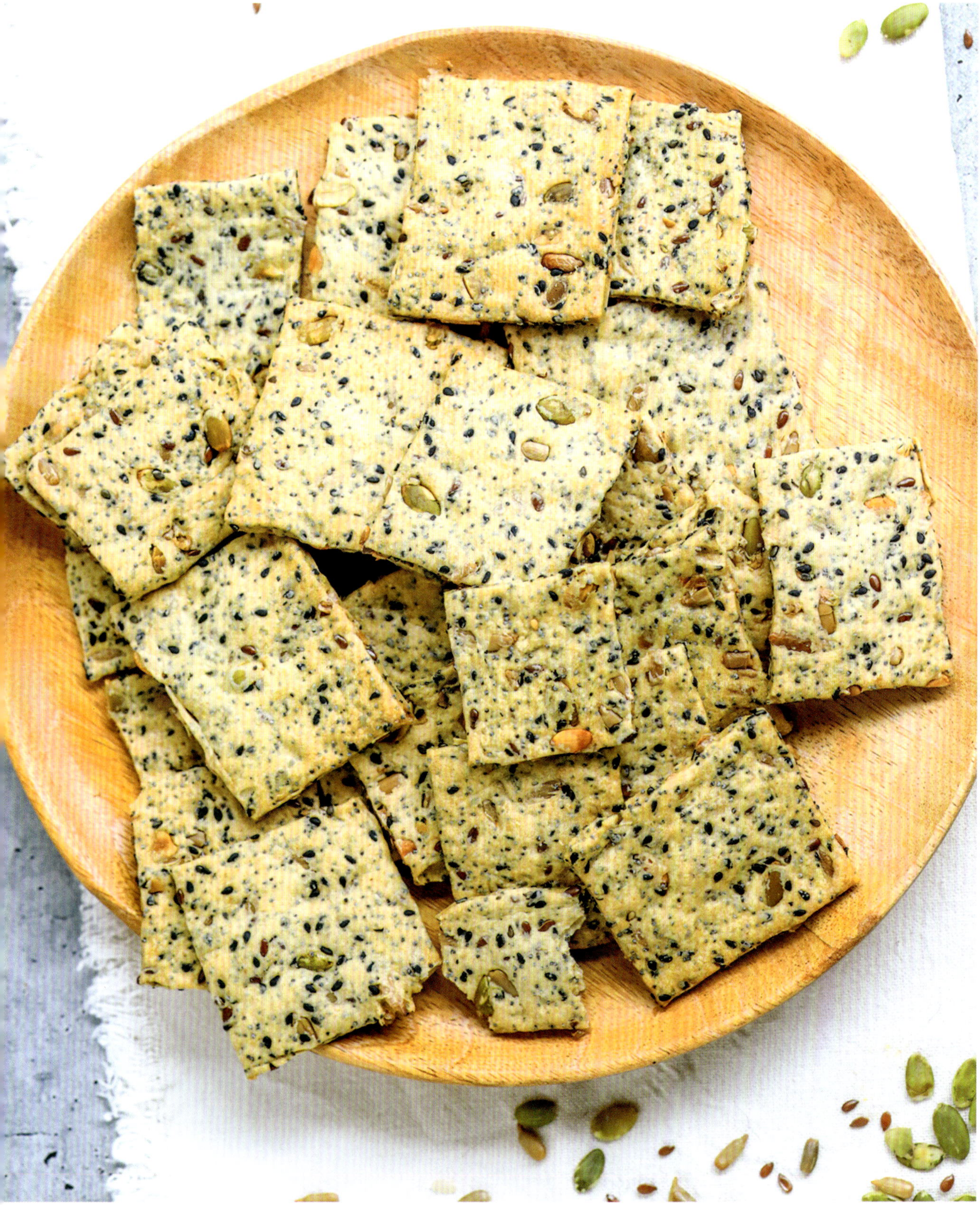

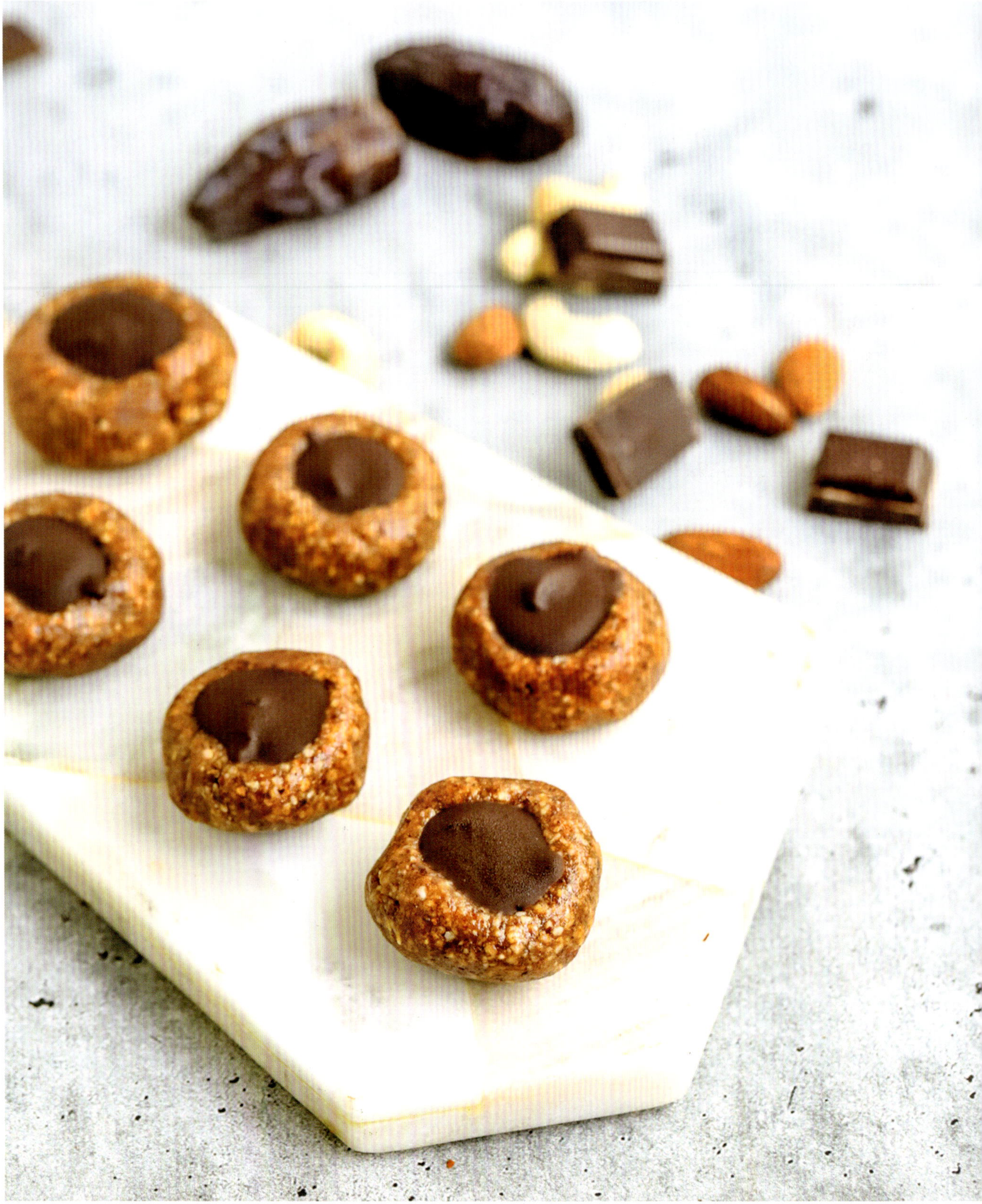

SERVES **8** | **10** MINUTES

NUT BITES

INGREDIENTS

1.8 oz (50 g) **roasted almonds**
2 tbsp **roasted cashews**
5.3 oz (150 g) **soft dates**, pitted
1.8 oz (50 g) **nut butter** of choice
1.8 oz (50 g) **dark chocolate**

METHOD

- Place the almonds and cashew nuts into a food processor and blend. Now add the dates and nut butter and blend to a dough like consistency.
- Shape the mixture into small portions, leaving a cavity in the middle of each. Melt the dark chocolate and pour it into the cavities.
- Place the bites into the refrigerator until set firm.

ENERGY: **34** Kcal	CARBS: **3** g	PROTEIN: **1** g	FAT: **2** g

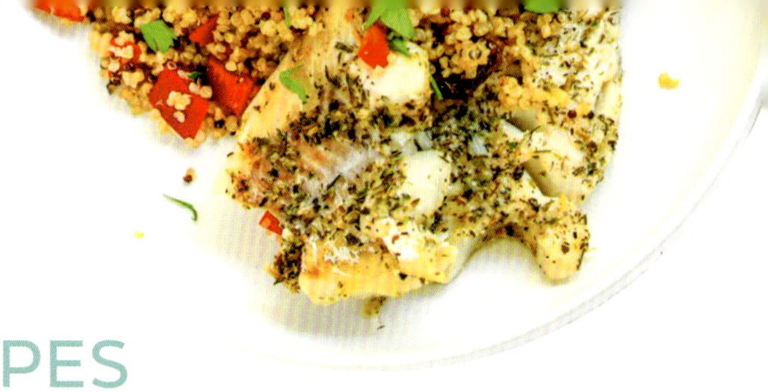

RECIPES WEEK 3

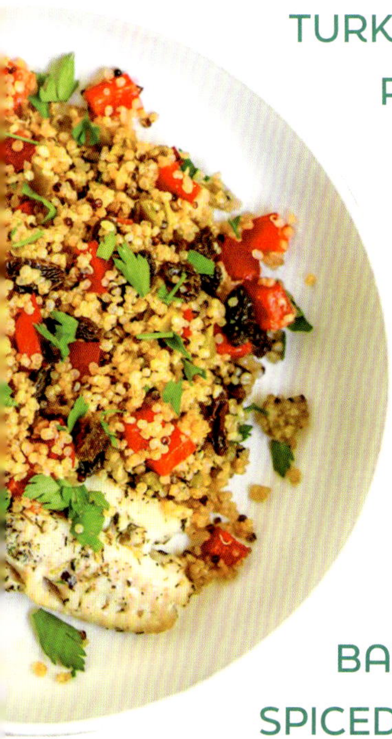

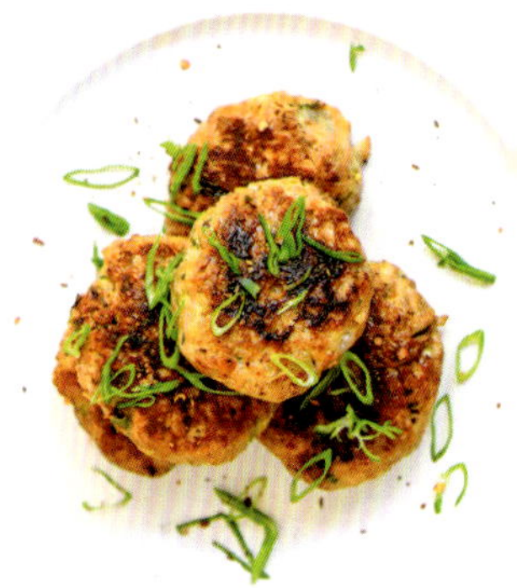

TURKEY AND GREEN ONION BREAKFAST PATTIES
PEACH AND PECAN PROTEIN SMOOTHIE
GREEN EGGS AND HAM TORTILLA
STOVE TOP BAKED BEANS
CHICKEN CRUST PIZZA
CHICKEN COLESLAW SALAD
SMASH BURGER TACOS
TUNA AVO RICE BOWL
KOREAN BEEF SALAD WRAPS
BAKED SALMON RICE WAFFLES
BAKED CHICKEN WITH LEMON-CHIVE SAUCE
SPICED HADDOCK WITH QUINOA AND RAISIN SALAD
SALTED CARAMEL COTTAGE CHEESE ICE CREAM
PROTEIN PEANUT BUTTER CUPS
KEFIR CHIA SEED PUDDING

WEEKLY SHOPPING LIST

PRODUCE

1 avocado
1 banana
blueberries
1 lemon
2 limes
2 peaches
3 onions
½ red onion
large bunch green onions (spring onions)
2 bulb garlic
root ginger
3 carrots
2 baby cucumbers
1 cucumber
1 orange bell pepper
1 jalapeño pepper
2 heads of lettuce spinach
red cabbage basil
chives
cilantro (coriander) parsley
6 medjool dates raisins

PROTEIN

1.2 lb (530 g) boneless, skinless chicken breast
2 lb (900 g) ground turkey (minced turkey)
1 lb (450 g) ground chicken (minced chicken)
1 lb (450 g) 95% lean ground beef (minced beef)
9.2 oz (260 g) beef steak
pack sliced ham
2 x 4.2 oz (120 g) salmon fillets
2 x 4.9 oz (140 g) haddock fillets
3 eggs almond milk
Greek yogurt
kefir
shredded mozzarella cheese
ball of mozzarella cheese
sliced cheese of choice
1.1 lb (505 g) cottage cheese

DRY GOODS

rolled oats
basmati rice
white rice
sushi rice
almonds
pecans
chia seeds
quinoa
sesame seeds
all-purpose flour
dark chocolate chips
vanilla extract
red pepper flakes (chili flakes)
paprika
smoked paprika
ground cinnamon
ground cumin
fennel seeds
garlic powder
Italian seasoning

STAPLES AND MISC

coconut oil
sesame oil
honey
maple syrup
1 x 14 oz (400 g) can cannellini beans
1 x 4.8 oz (135 g) can tuna
natural peanut butter
tamari sauce
kecap
manis
tomato ketchup
tomato paste (purée)
sieved tomatoes (tomato passata)
barbecue sauce
Worcestershire sauce
hot sauce
rice wine vinegar
Dijon mustard
mayonnaise
dill pickles (gherkins)
kimchi
whole wheat tortillas
small corn tortillas
breadcrumbs
nori
vanilla protein powder

Sample Weekly Meal Planner

	BREAKFAST	LUNCH
Monday	TURKEY AND GREEN ONION BREAKFAST PATTIES	CHICKEN CRUST PIZZA
Tueday	TURKEY AND GREEN ONION BREAKFAST PATTIES	KOREAN BEEF SALAD WRAPS
Wednesday	GREEN EGGS AND HAM TORTILLA	CHICKEN COLESLAW SALAD
Thursday	STOVE TOP BAKED BEANS	CHICKEN COLESLAW SALAD
Friday	STOVE TOP BAKED BEANS	SMASH BURGER TACOS
Saturday	GREEN EGGS AND HAM TORTILLA	SMASH BURGER TACOS
Sunday	PEACH AND PECAN PROTEIN SMOOTHIE	CHICKEN CRUST PIZZA

SNACK	DINNER
PROTEIN PEANUT BUTTER CUPS	KOREAN BEEF SALAD WRAPS
PROTEIN PEANUT BUTTER CUPS	TUNA AVO RICE BOWL
KEFIR CHIA SEED PUDDING	BAKED SALMON RICE WAFFLES
KEFIR CHIA SEED PUDDING	BAKED CHICKEN WITH LEMON-CHIVE SAUCE
PROTEIN PEANUT BUTTER CUPS	BAKED CHICKEN WITH LEMON-CHIVE SAUCE
SALTED CARAMEL COTTAGE CHEESE ICE CREAM	MEAL OUT – ENJOY!
SALTED CARAMEL COTTAGE CHEESE ICE CREAM	SPICED HADDOCK WITH QUINOA AND RAISIN SALAD

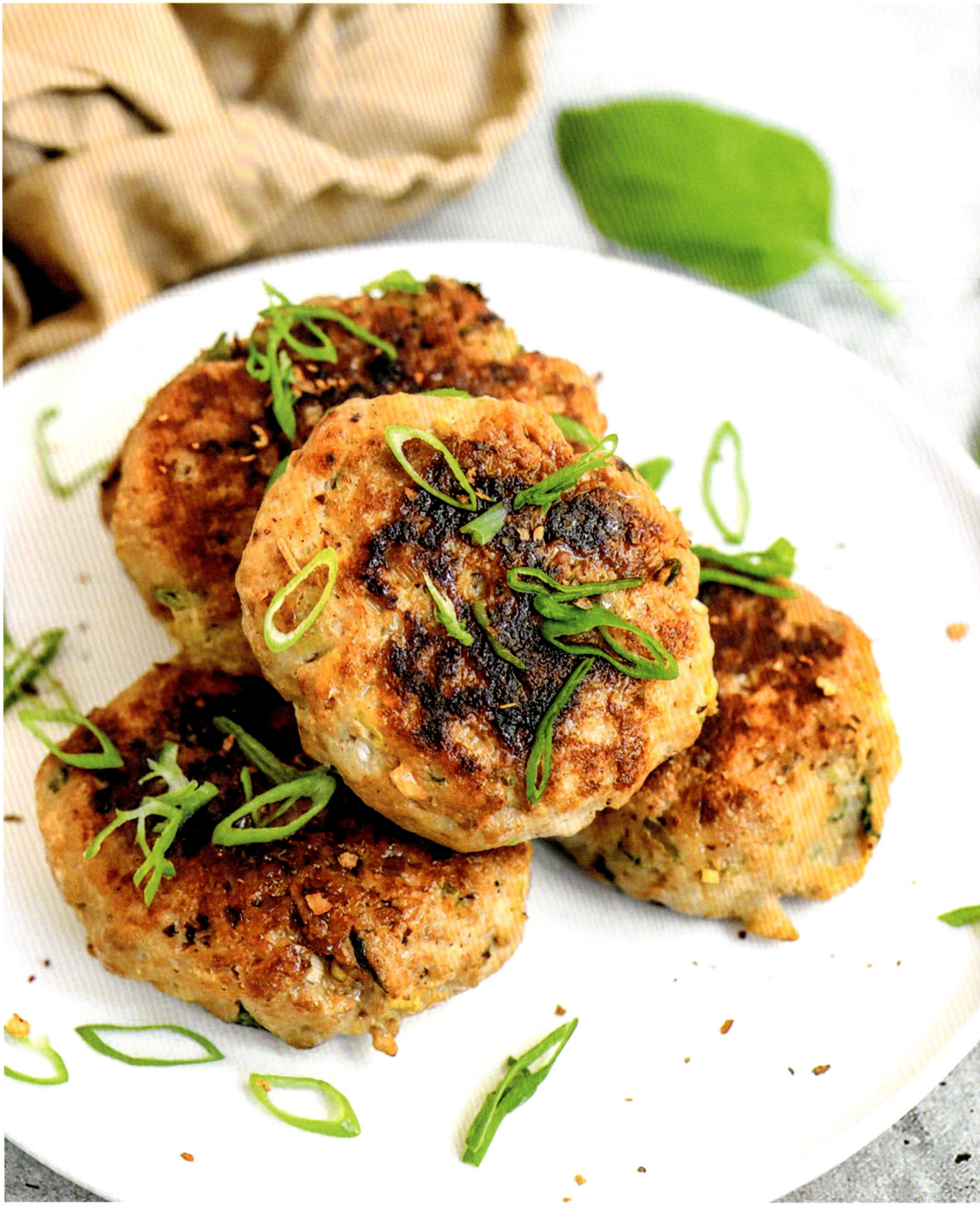

TURKEY AND GREEN ONION BREAKFAST PATTIES

INGREDIENTS

2 lb (900 g) **ground turkey**
1 tbsp **tamari sauce**
2 tsp **ginger**, freshly grated
3 tbsp **green onions**, minced
4 **garlic** cloves, minced
½ tsp **red pepper** flakes
6 **basil leaves**, minced
1½ tsp **sea salt**
2 tbsp **extra virgin olive oil**

METHOD

- In a large bowl, combine the ground turkey with the tamari sauce, ginger, green onions, garlic, red pepper flakes, basil and salt. Mix well, then with wet hands, form the mixture into 16 even-sized patties and flatten them gently between your two hands until about ½" (1 cm) thick.
- Heat the olive oil in a large skillet over medium heat. Working in batches, add the patties to the skillet, and cook on both sides until the patties have browned, this will take around 6–8 minutes. Continue cooking, occasionally flipping the patties over, for a further 4–6 minutes. Repeat this process with remaining patties.
- Storage: Once cooked and cooled, leftover patties can be stored in an airtight container in the refrigerator for up to 5 days, or in the freezer for up to 1 month.

ENERGY: **201** Kcal | CARBS: **0** g | PROTEIN: **21** g | FAT: **13** g

SERVES **1** | **5** MINUTES

PEACH AND PECAN PROTEIN SMOOTHIE

INGREDIENTS

6 fl oz (180 ml) **almond milk**, unsweetened
5.8 oz (165 g) **Greek yogurt**
1 **peach**, chopped, frozen
½ **banana**
0.5 oz (15 g) **pecans**
2 tbsp **rolled oats**
¼ tsp **vanilla extract**
¼ tsp **ground cinnamon**
pinch of **sea salt**

METHOD

- Place all the ingredients into a high speed blender and blitz until smooth. Pour into a glass and serve immediately.

ENERGY: **434** Kcal	CARBS: **46** g	PROTEIN: **22** g	FAT: **18** g

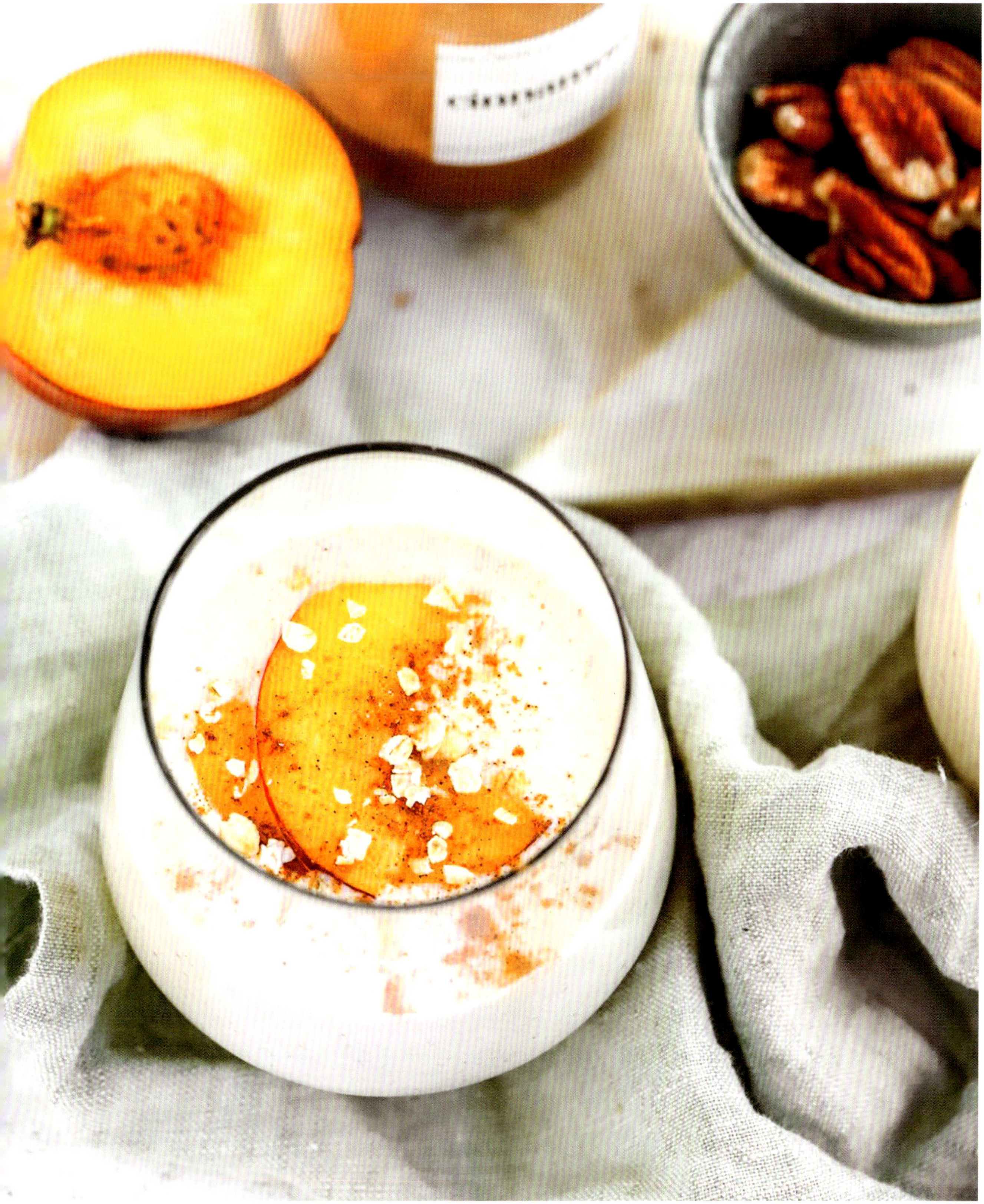

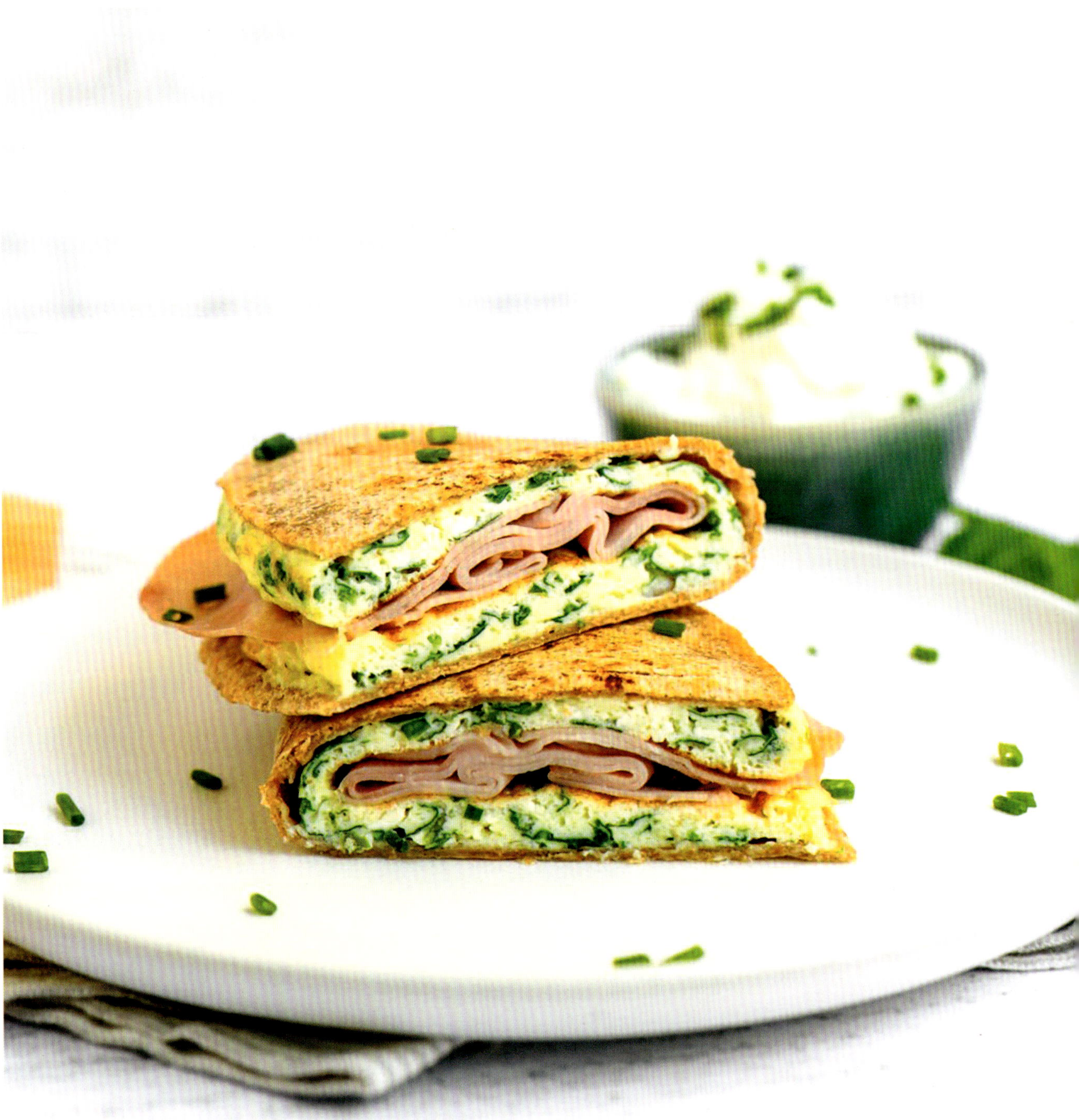

SERVES **1** | **10** MINUTES

GREEN EGGS AND HAM TORTILLA

INGREDIENTS

2 **eggs**
1 **green onion**, sliced
handful **spinach**, chopped
1.9 oz (55 g) **cottage cheese**
whole wheat tortilla
2.1 oz (60 g) sliced **ham**

METHOD

- In a bowl, whisk together the eggs, onion, spinach and cottage cheese. Season with salt and pepper.
- Preheat a non-stick skillet over medium-high heat. Add the egg mixture to the skillet and top with the tortilla. Cook for 3–4 minutes, or until the eggs are cooked to your preference.
- Using a plate to cover the skillet, flip the skillet upside down so the tortilla goes onto the plate. Then slide the tortilla back into the pan with the eggs facing up.
- Top the eggs with the ham and fold the tortilla in two. Slice the tortilla in half and serve immediately.

ENERGY: **403** Kcal	CARBS: **23** g	PROTEIN: **35** g	FAT: **19** g

STOVE TOP BAKED BEANS

INGREDIENTS

1 tbsp **olive oil**
2 **onions**, diced
2 tbsp **tomato ketchup**
1 tbsp **tomato purée**
2 tbsp **barbecue sauce**
2 tsp **Worcestershire sauce**
1 tsp **Dijon mustard**
1 tbsp **maple syrup**
½ tsp smoked **paprika**
½ tsp **ground cumin**
14 oz (400 g) can **cannellini beans**, drained
3.4 fl oz (100 ml) **water**

METHOD

- Heat the olive oil in a pot and sauté the onions on low-medium heat for about 5 minutes.
- In a small bowl, mix together the tomato ketchup, tomato purée, barbecue sauce, Worcestershire sauce, mustard, maple syrup, smoked paprika, cumin, salt and pepper. Add the sauce to the onions and mix well.
- Now add the beans and water to the onion mixture and stir until well combined. Simmer the beans for 10 minutes, until the water has reduced. Check for seasoning and add more salt and pepper as required.
- Serve the beans with bread or toast (not included in nutritional breakdown).

ENERGY: 267 Kcal | CARBS: 45 g | PROTEIN: 6 g | FAT: 7 g

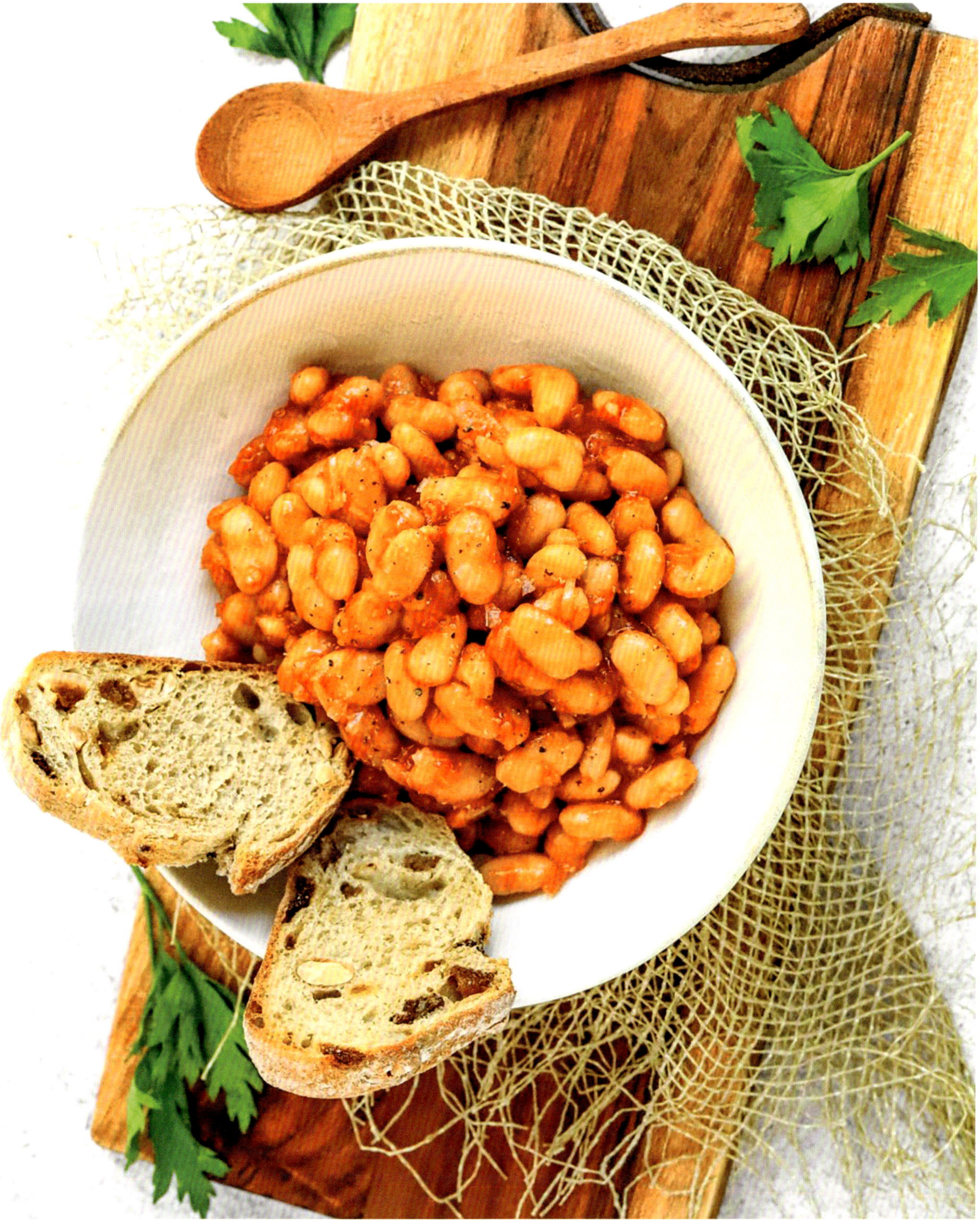

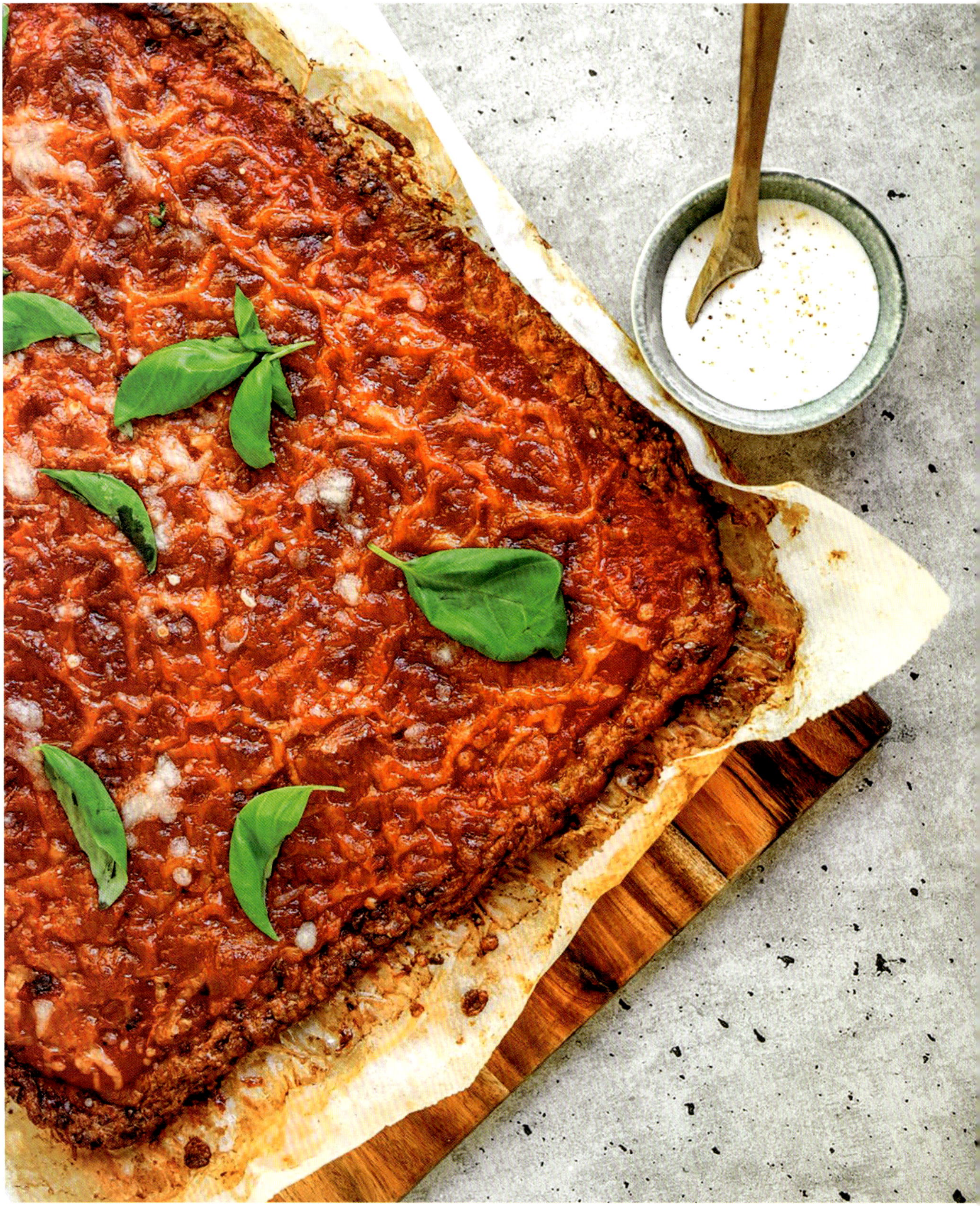

SERVES **4** | **35** MINUTES

CHICKEN CRUST **PIZZA**

INGREDIENTS

1 lb (450 g) **ground chicken**
2 oz (57 g) **mozzarella cheese**, shredded
1 tsp **Italian seasoning**
¼ tsp **sea salt**

Pizza toppings

2 fl oz (120 ml) **passata**
1 **mozzarella ball**, sliced
handful **basil** leaves

METHOD

- Preheat the oven to 400°F (200°C). Line a baking sheet with baking paper, or a silicone baking mat.
- Add the ground chicken, cheese, Italian seasoning and salt to a bowl and mix thoroughly with your hands.
- Place the mixture on the prepared baking sheet and spread into a pizza shape about ¼" (½cm) thick. Place into the preheated oven to bake for 20 minutes. If any liquid leaks out of the crust, absorb with kitchen towels.
- Remove from the oven and spread the passata on top, then add the mozzarella cheese and bake for a further 10 minutes until the cheese has melted.
- Remove from the oven and cool slightly, before topping with fresh basil leaves, slicing and serving.

ENERGY: **267** Kcal | CARBS: **2** g | PROTEIN: **28** g | FAT: **17** g

SERVES **2** | **22** MINUTES

CHICKEN COLESLAW SALAD

INGREDIENTS

8.1 oz (230 g) **boneless**, skinless chicken breast
2 tbsp **olive oil**
2 tbsp **lime juice**
1 tbsp **tamari sauce**
1 tsp **honey**
½ tsp **red pepper** flakes
6 oz (170 g) **red cabbage**, shredded
2 **carrots**, grated
2 **green onions**, sliced
2 tbsp **cilantro**, chopped
1.4 oz (40 g) **roasted almonds**, chopped

METHOD

- Add the chicken to a pot and cover with 1" (2.5 cm) of water. Bring to a boil then reduce the heat to a medium-low.
- Partially cover the pot with a lid and simmer for 10–12 minutes, or until the chicken is cooked through. Place the cooked chicken into a bowl and shred it with two forks. Set aside to cool.
- Meanwhile, place the olive oil, lime juice, tamari, honey and red pepper flakes in a large bowl, and whisk until well combined.
- Now add the cabbage, carrots, green onions, cilantro and almonds to the bowls and toss gently to ensure all the ingredients are well coated in the dressing. Stir in the chicken and stir again.
- Divide the salad equally between 2 bowls or plates and serve.

ENERGY: **455** Kcal	CARBS: **21** g	PROTEIN: **32** g	FAT: **27** g

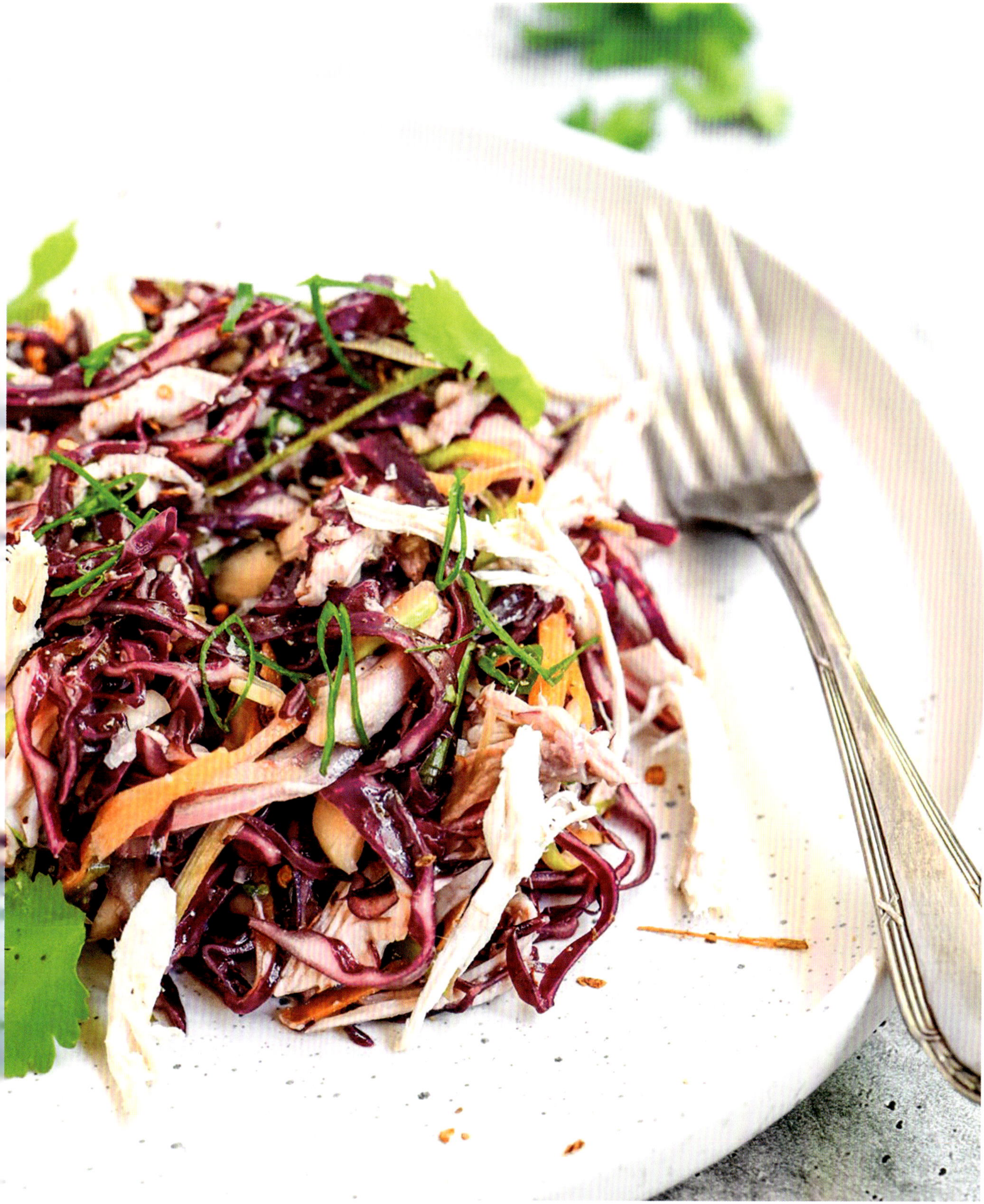

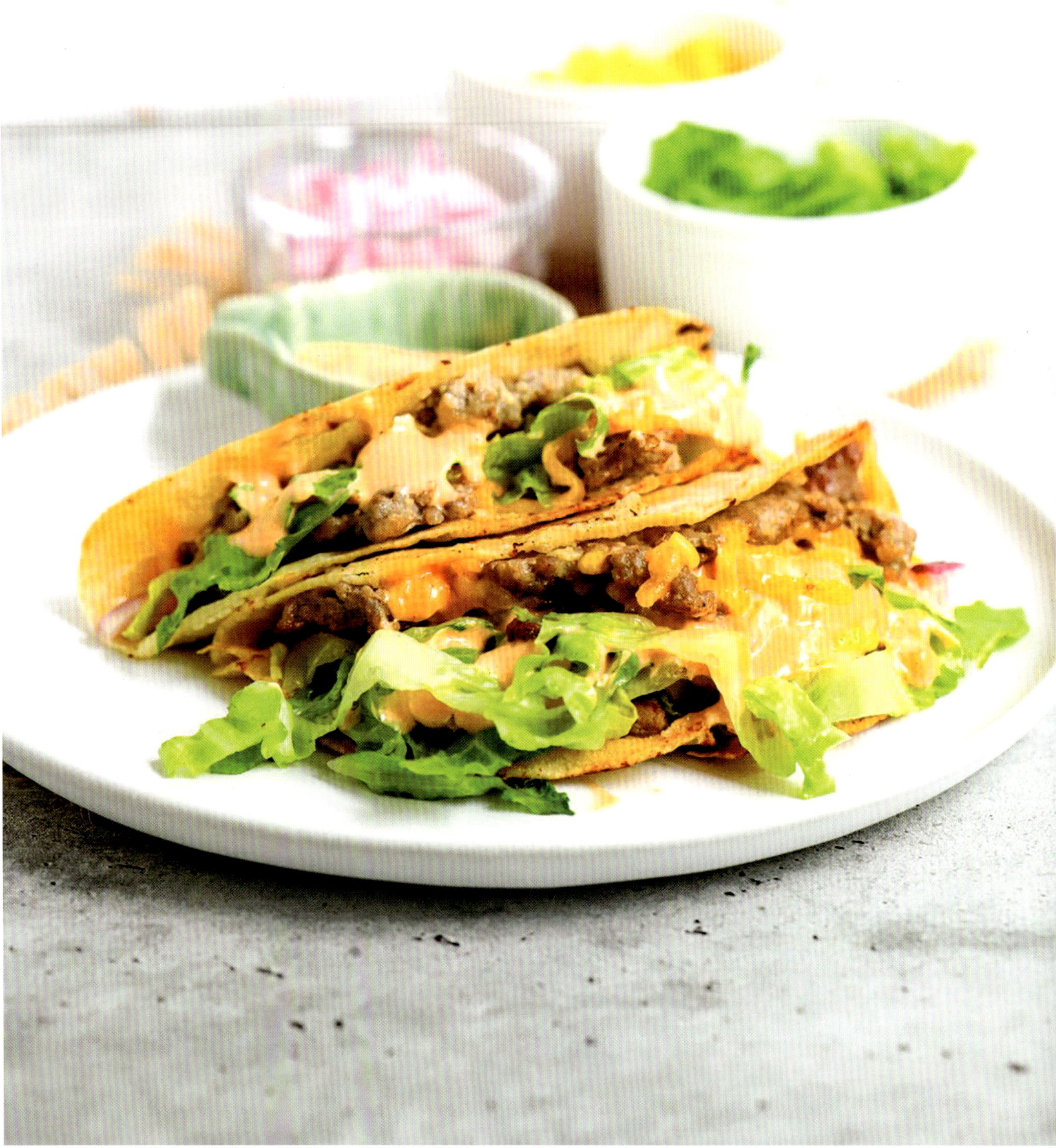

SERVES **4** | **20** MINUTES

SMASH BURGER **TACOS**

INGREDIENTS

4 tbsp **mayonnaise**
1 tbsp **tomato ketchup**
1 tsp **Dijon mustard**
1–2 **dill pickles**, diced
½ tsp **hot sauce**
1 lb (450 g) **95% ground beef**
1 tsp **sea salt**
½ tsp ground **black pepper**
4 (6"/15 cm) **corn tortillas**
1 slice **cheese**, cut in half lengthwise
2.7 oz (75 g) **shredded lettuce**
1.2 oz (35 g) **onions**, diced

METHOD

- Place the mayonnaise, tomato ketchup, mustard, dill pickles and hot sauce in a small bowl, stir to combine and set aside.
- Heat a skillet over medium-high heat.
- Season the beef with salt and pepper and divide into 4 even-sized portions. Form burgers with your hands, then place on the hot pan and cook for 2 minutes. Place a tortilla on top of each beef burger and press down to flatten the beef into the shape and size of the tortilla.
- Cook for a further 2–3 minutes, until the tortilla is golden brown. Flip each patty over and top with cheese. Once the cheese has melted, and the tortilla has lightly browned, top with lettuce and onions.
- Drizzle with the sauce, then remove from the skillet and fold in half like a taco. Serve immediately.

ENERGY: **411** Kcal | CARBS: **14** g | PROTEIN: **28** g | FAT: **27** g

SERVES **2** | **10** MINUTES

TUNA AVO RICE BOWL

INGREDIENTS

4.8 oz (135 g) can **tuna**, drained
½ **avocado**
4 tbsp **red onion**, finely diced
½ **lemon**, juiced
1 tsp **red pepper flakes**
½ tsp **fennel seeds**
1 tbsp **mayonnaise**
¼ tsp **sea salt**
6.3 oz (180 g) **cooked white rice**
2 **baby cucumbers**, finely chopped
½ **carrot**, grated
4 tbsp **chives**, finely chopped
2 tbsp **nori**, chopped

METHOD

- Add the drained tuna, avocado, onion, lemon juice, red pepper flakes, fennel seeds, mayonnaise and salt into a bowl and mash with a fork to combine.
- Mix in the cooked rice, cucumbers, carrots and chives.
- Divide the mixture evenly between 2 bowls and top with the nori.

ENERGY: **365** kcal | CARBS: **39** g | PROTEIN: **23** g | FAT: **13** g

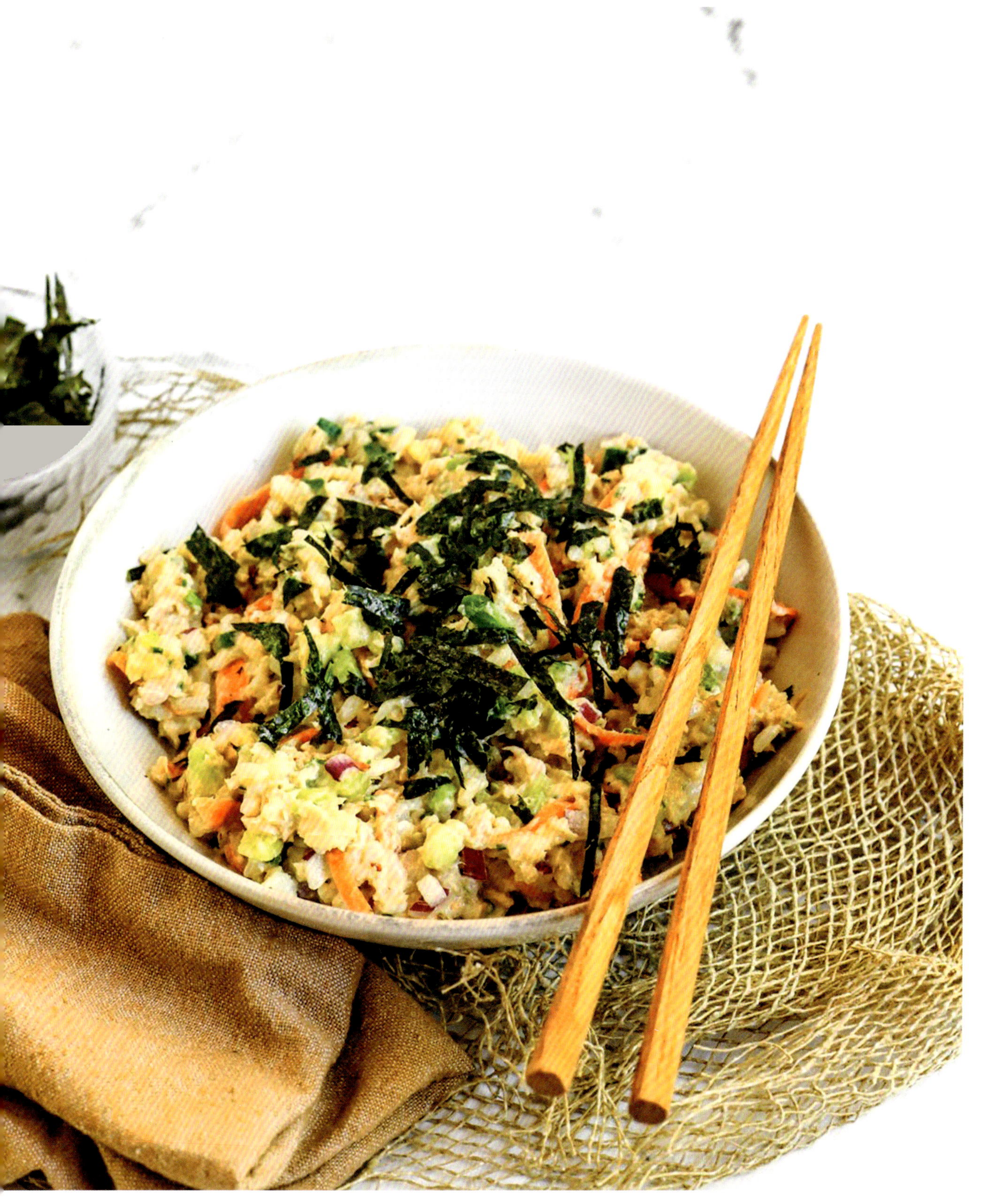

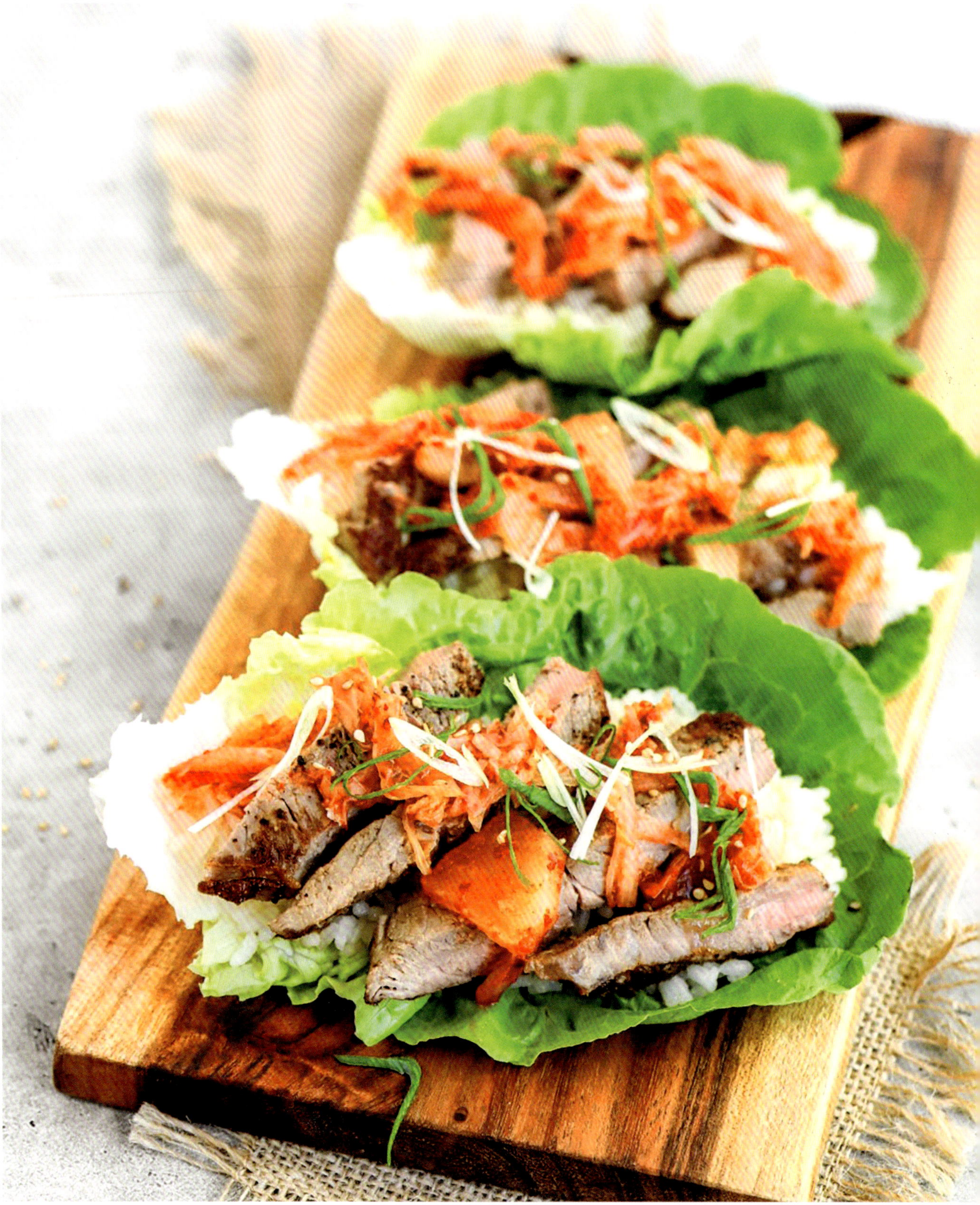

SERVES **2** | **25** MINUTES

KOREAN BEEF SALAD WRAPS

INGREDIENTS

3.5 oz (100 g) **basmati rice**
4 tbsp **sesame oil**
9.2 oz (260 g) **beef steak**
8 **lettuce leaves**
6 tbsp **kimchi**

METHOD

- Cook the rice according to package instructions.
- Heat the sesame oil in a skillet and sauté the steaks for 2 minutes on each side, until cooked to medium. Season with salt and pepper to taste and cut into strips.
- Fill the lettuce leaves with a layer of cooked rice, followed by beef strips, then top with kimchi and serve.

ENERGY: **388** kcal	CARBS: **20** g	PROTEIN: **4** g	FAT: **28** g

SERVES **2** | **35** MINUTES

BAKED SALMON RICE **WAFFLES**

INGREDIENTS

2 x 4.2 oz (120 g) **salmon fillets**
2 tbsp **kecap manis**
6.4 oz (180 g) **cooked sushi rice**
1 tsp **rice wine vinegar**
½ tsp **sesame oil**
1 **cucumber**, finely sliced
½ **avocado**, mashed
2 tbsp **mayonnaise**
2 tbsp **hot sauce**
1 tsp **sesame seeds**
½ **lime**, juiced

METHOD

- Preheat the oven to 355°F (180°C). Line a baking sheet with baking paper.
- Coat the salmon with the kecap manis, place onto the baking sheet and bake in the hot oven for 15 minutes, or until cooked through.
- Cook the sushi rice according to packet instructions, once cooked mix in the rice wine vinegar and sesame oil.
- Pack the rice into a waffle maker on the highest heat setting and cook for 8 minutes, or until the rice is crispy and slightly browned. Make sure the waffle maker is very full with the rice and press firmly so that it sticks together to form the waffle shape.
- Once the salmon is cooked, flake the salmon into bite size pieces using a fork.
- Top the crispy rice waffles with the cucumber, avocado, salmon, mayonnaise, hot sauce of choice, sesame seeds and a drizzle over the lime juice.

ENERGY: **475** kcal | CARBS: **47** g | PROTEIN: **20** g | FAT: **23** g

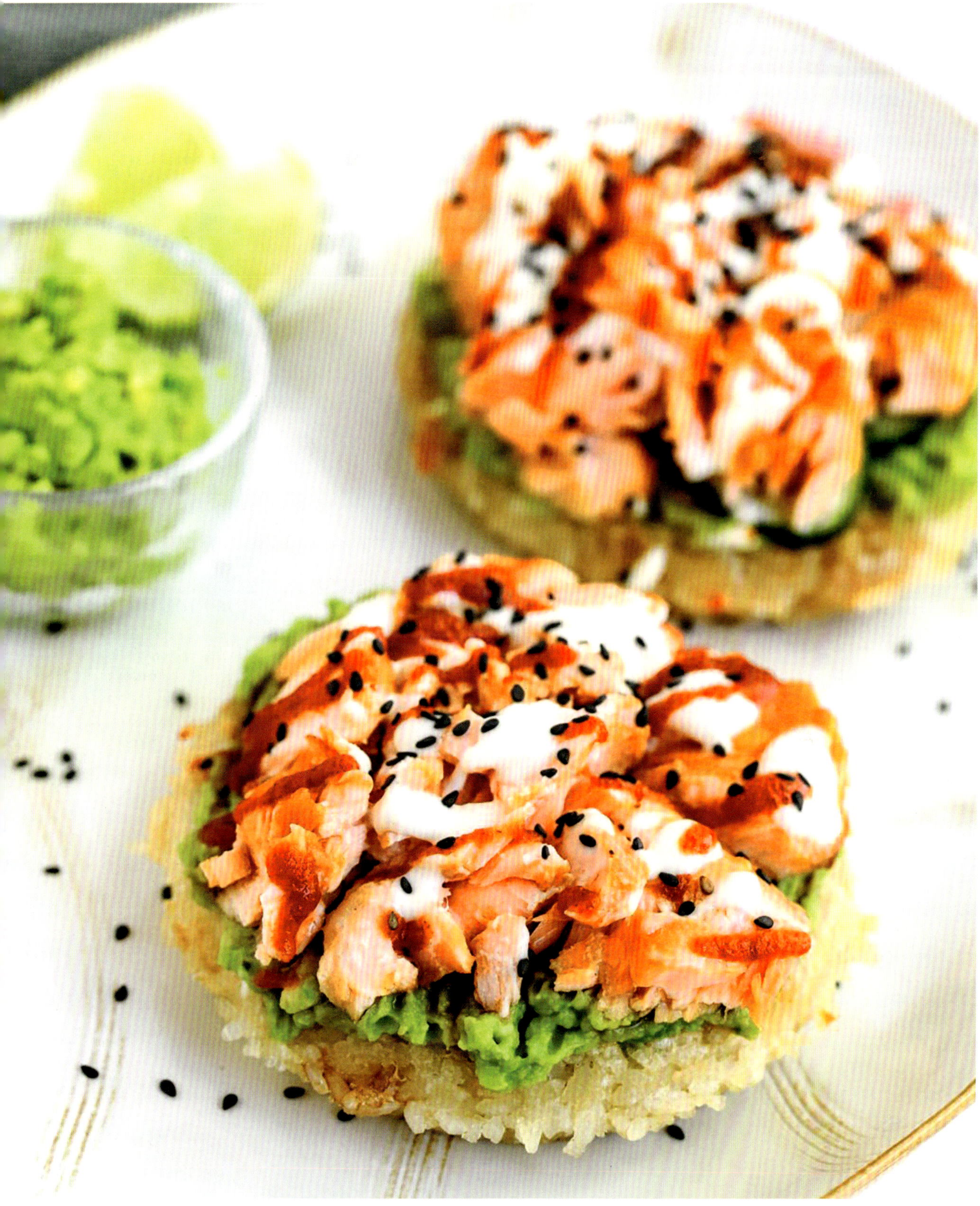

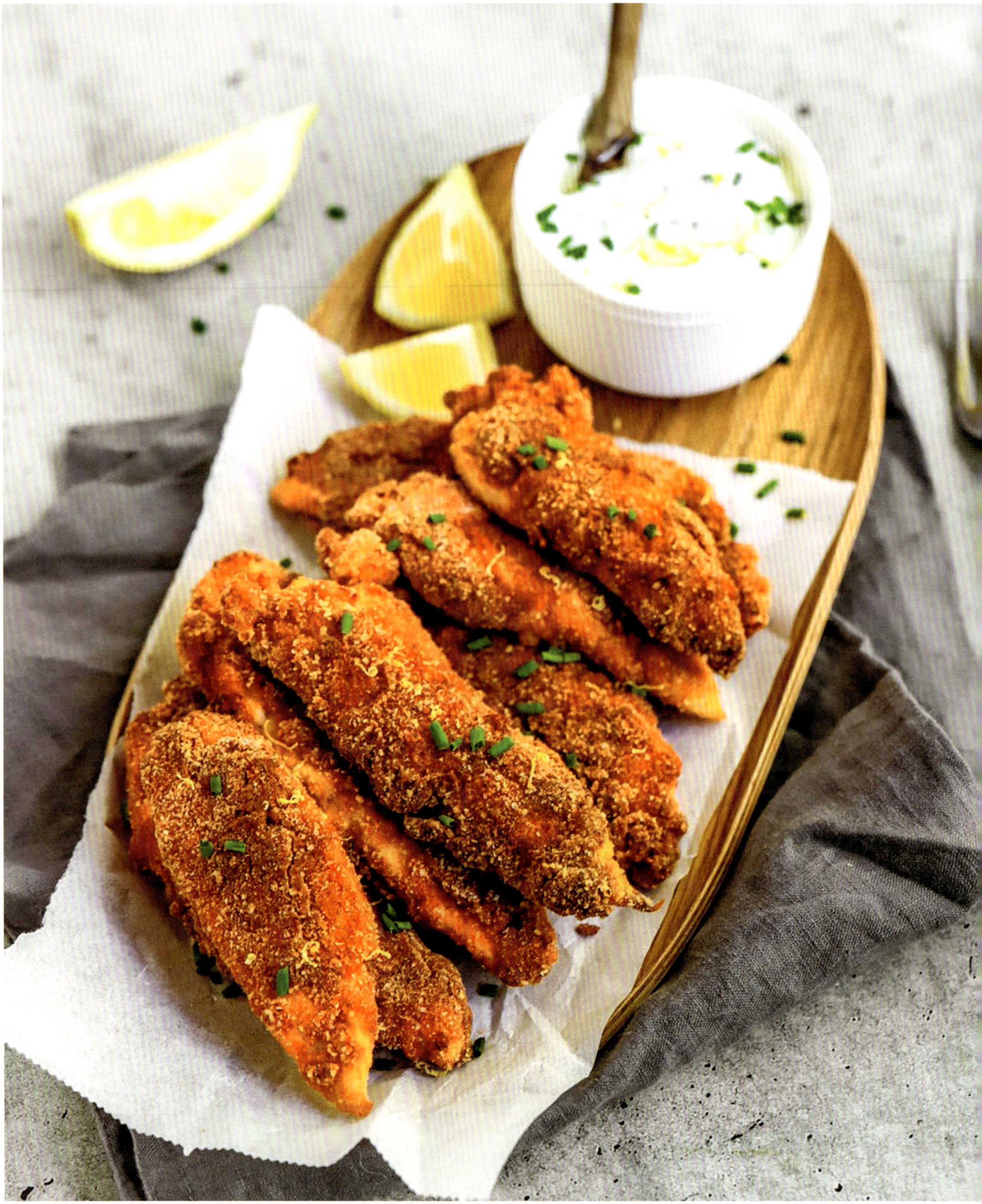

SERVES **2** | **30** MINUTES

BAKED CHICKEN WITH LEMON-CHIVE SAUCE

INGREDIENTS

For the chicken

10.6 oz (300 g) **boneless**, skinless chicken breasts
1 **egg**
2 tbsp **olive oil**
1 tbsp **paprika**
1 tbsp **garlic powder**
0.7 oz (20 g) **all-purpose flour**
2.1 oz (60 g) **breadcrumbs**

For the sauce

2 tbsp **chives**, chopped
3.5 oz (100 g) **Greek yogurt**
½ **lemon**, juice and zest

METHOD

- Preheat the oven to 400°F (200°C). Line a baking sheet with baking paper.
- Cut the chicken breasts into bite-sized strips.
- Crack the egg into a bowl and whisk together with 1 tablespoon of the olive oil, salt, pepper, paprika and garlic powder.
- First cover chicken into the flour, then into the egg and spice mixture, and finally into the breadcrumbs.
- Place the chicken onto the baking sheet and drizzle over the remaining tablespoon of olive oil. Place the baking sheet into the hot oven and bake the chicken for 7 minutes.
- Remove from the oven and flip the chicken pieces over and bake for a further 10 minutes until the chicken is golden and cooked through.
- Meanwhile, place the chives, Greek yogurt, lemon juice and ½ of the lemon zest into a bowl, season with salt and pepper and whisk to combine.
- Serve the chicken immediately, with the lemon-chive dipping sauce. Serve with green salad.

ENERGY: **555** kcal | CARBS: **39** g | PROTEIN: **48** g | FAT: **23** g

SERVES **2** | **30** MINUTES

SPICED HADDOCK WITH QUINOA AND RAISIN SALAD

INGREDIENTS

3 oz (85 g) **dry quinoa**
2 x 4.9 oz (140 g) **haddock fillets**
1 tsp **Italian seasoning**
1 tbsp **olive oil**
½ **jalapeño pepper**, diced
½ **orange bell pepper**, diced
1.8 oz (50 g) **raisins**
½ **lime**, juiced
1 tbsp **parsley**, chopped, to garnish

METHOD

- Cook the quinoa according to the package directions. Drain and set aside.
- Season the fillets all over with the Italian seasoning, salt, and pepper.
- Heat half of the olive oil in a skillet over medium heat. Cook the haddock for around 5 minutes on each side or until the fish is cooked through.
- In a bowl, mix together the quinoa, jalapeño, bell pepper and raisins. Add the remaining olive oil and lime juice, mix well and season with salt and pepper.
- Divide the fish and quinoa evenly between 2 plates. Top with a garnish of parsley and serve immediately.

ENERGY: **450** kcal | CARBS: **52** g | PROTEIN: **38** g | FAT: **10** g

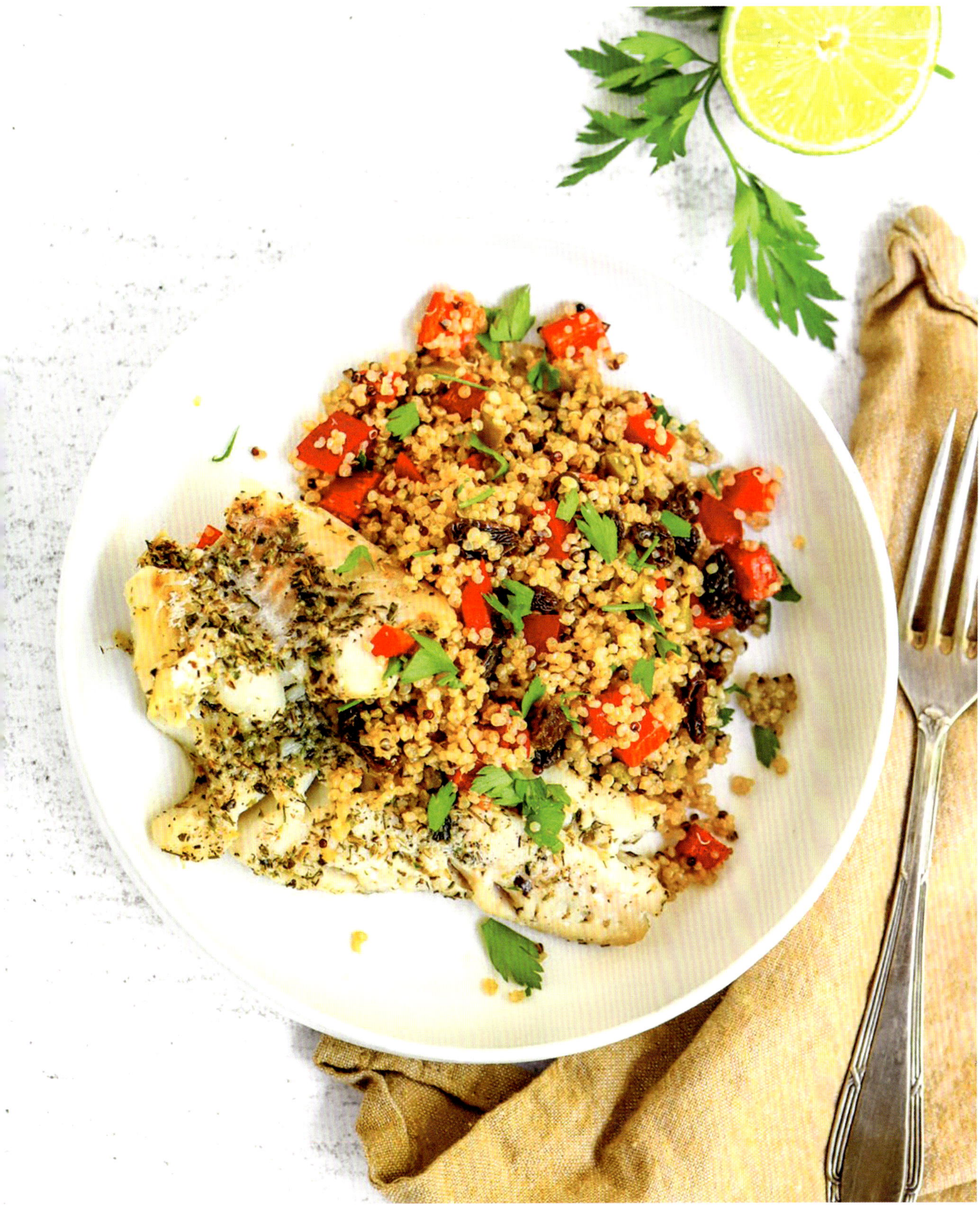

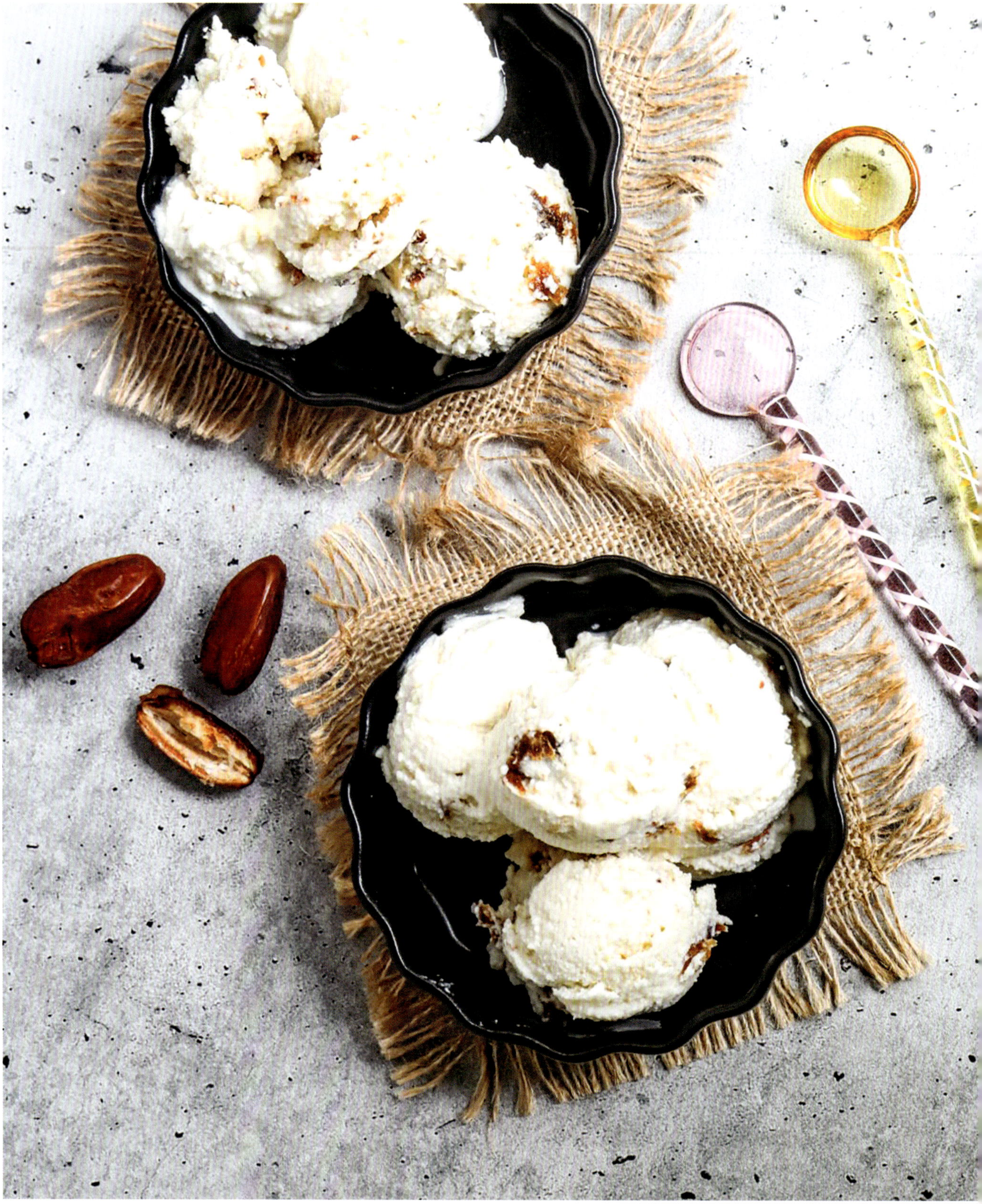

SERVES **4** | **4** HOURS **5** MINUTES

SALTED CARAMEL COTTAGE CHEESE ICE CREAM

INGREDIENTS

1 lb (450 g) **cottage cheese**
4 tbsp **honey**
½ tsp **vanilla extract**
pinch of **sea salt**
6 **medjool dates**

METHOD

- Add the cottage cheese, honey, vanilla extract and sea salt to a food processor or blender. Blend until smooth, then add the dates and blend again. You want the dates to be broken up but not fully blended.
- Add the mixture to a freezer proof dish, or loaf pan, and freeze for 3–4 hours until ice cream has set.
- Before serving, remove from the freezer and set aside to rest for 10–15 minutes.

ENERGY: **289** kcal	CARBS: **48** g	PROTEIN: **13** g	FAT: **5** g

SERVES **6** | **40** MINUTES

PROTEIN PEANUT BUTTER CUPS

INGREDIENTS

3 oz (85 g) **dark chocolate chips** (dairy-free if required)
2 tsp **coconut oil**
1 tbsp **almond milk**
4.4 oz (125 g) **natural peanut butter**
1 oz (30 g) **vanilla protein powder**
½ tsp **vanilla extract**

METHOD

- Place the coconut oil and chocolate chips into a small pot and melt over low heat. Remove from the heat before the chocolate chips have fully melted.
- Meanwhile, mix together the almond milk, peanut butter, protein powder and vanilla extract. Press the peanut butter mixture into mini silicone muffin moulds. Make sure to press down hard so that the mixture sticks together.
- Pour the melted chocolate over the top, dividing the chocolate equally between each peanut butter cup. Place into the freezer to set.

ENERGY: **246** kcal | CARBS: **11** g | PROTEIN: **10** g | FAT: **18** g

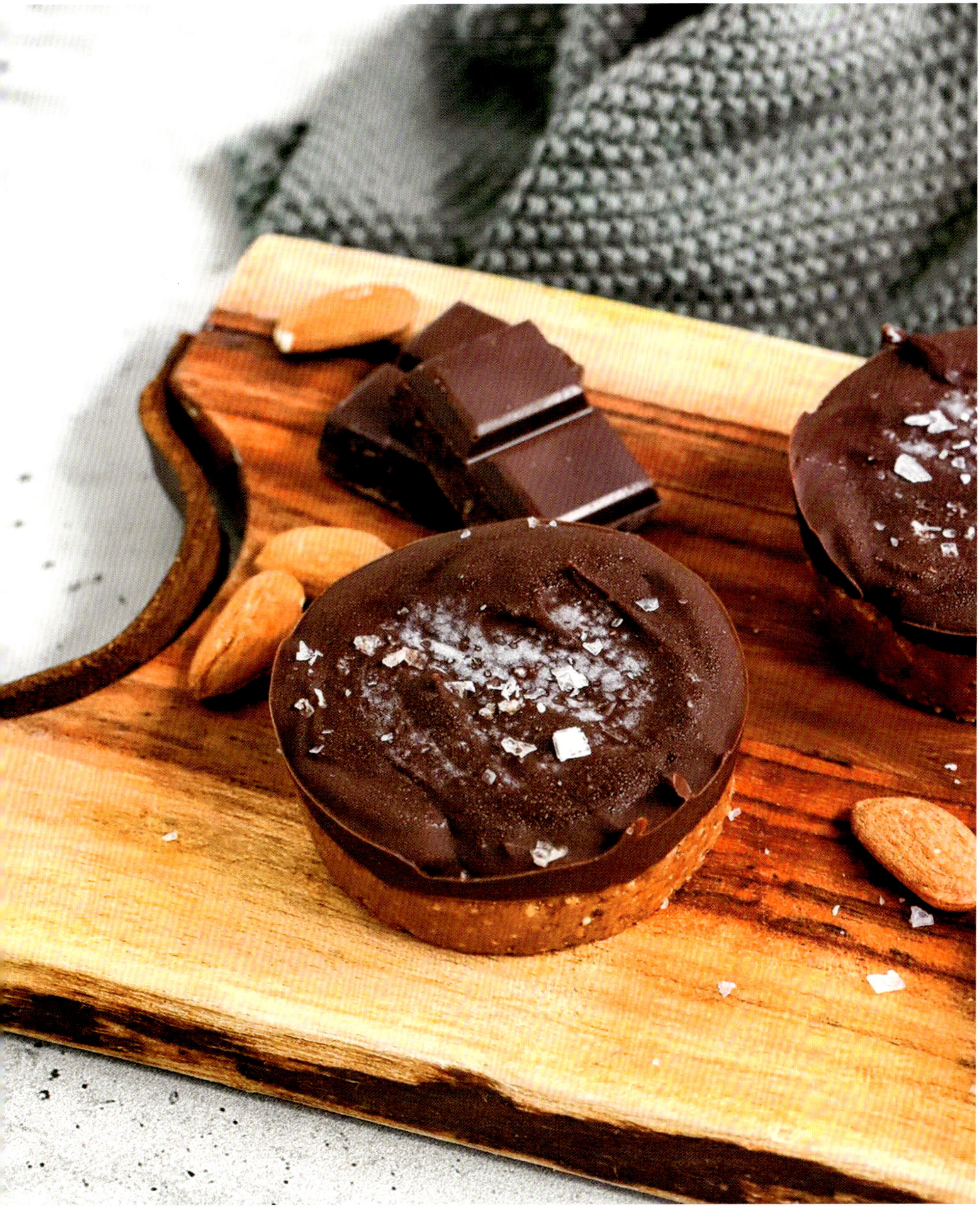

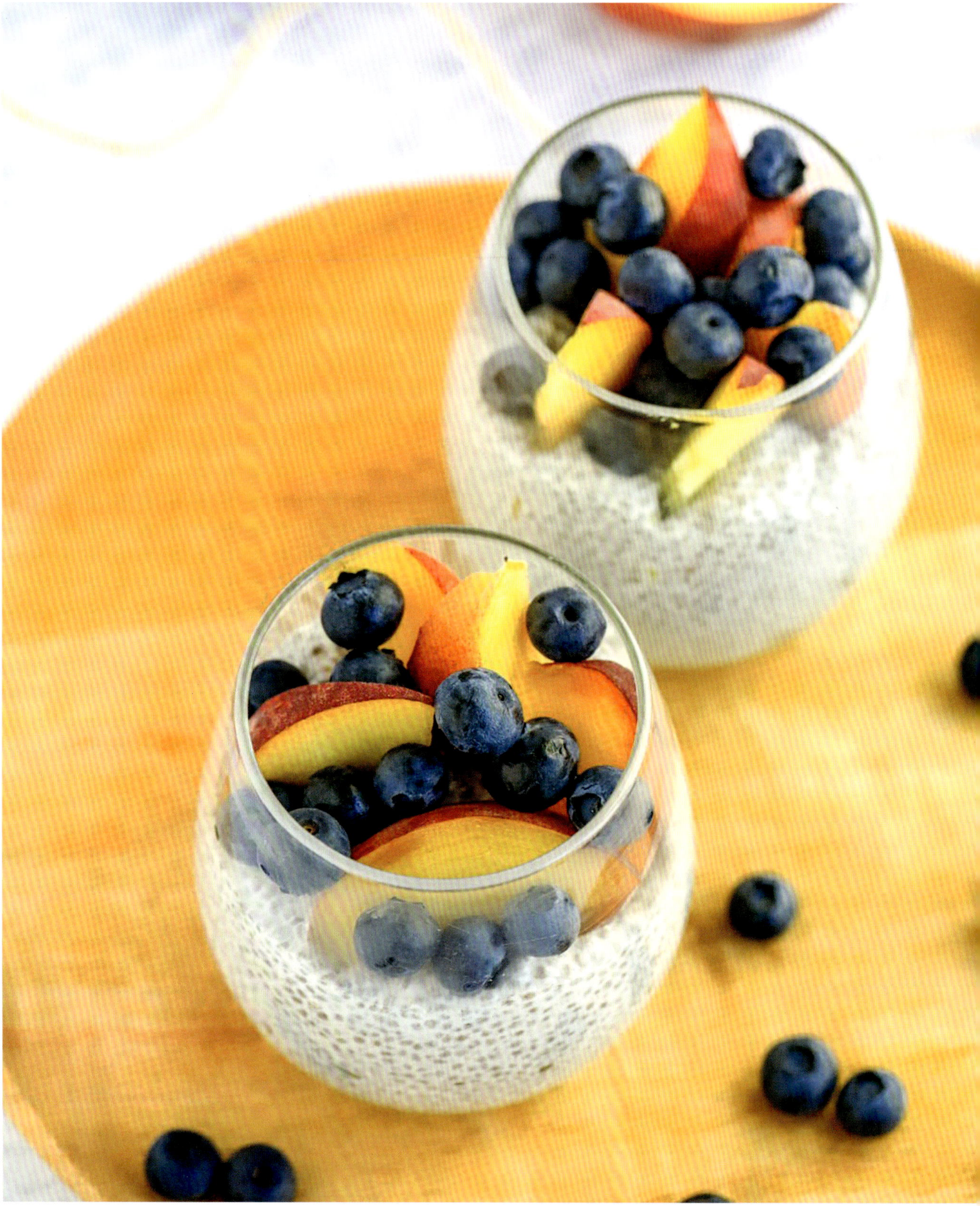

SERVES **3** | **2** HOURS **10** MINUTES

KEFIR CHIA SEED **PUDDING**

INGREDIENTS

9 tbsp **chia seeds**
1 tsp **ground cinnamon**
1.5 pints (720 ml) **kefir**
1 tbsp **maple syrup**
2.8 oz (80 g) **blueberries**
1 **peach**, diced

METHOD

- In a large jar or bowl, mix the chia seeds with the ground cinnamon.
- In a separate bowl or measuring cup, mix the kefir with the maple syrup.
- Pour the kefir mixture over the chia seeds and stir together until well combined. Cover and refrigerate for 2 hours or overnight.
- Once the mixture has become a pudding-like texture, remove from the fridge. Give everything a good stir, then portion into jars or bowls.
- When ready to serve, divide the blueberries and peaches equally over each of the puddings.

ENERGY: **386** kcal | CARBS: **46** g | PROTEIN: **19** g | FAT: **14** g

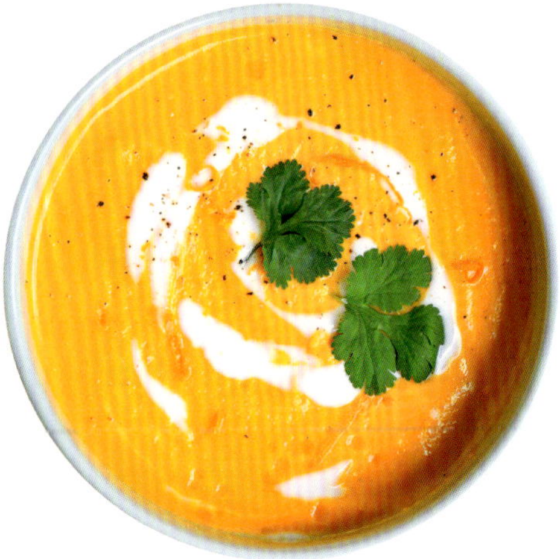

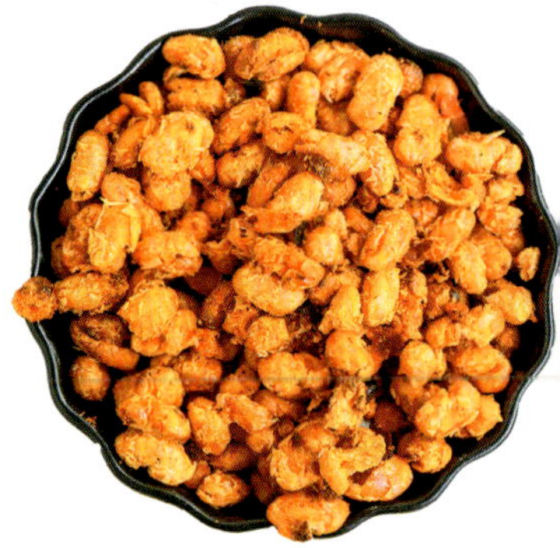

RECIPES WEEK 4

CHOCOLATE ALMOND DATE SMOOTHIE
VEGAN TOMATO AND MUSHROOM PANCAKES
VEGAN SOBRASADA (SAUSAGE SPREAD FROM MALLORCA)
TAHINI GRANOLA
JAPANESE CURRY UDON
CARROT SOUP
GREEN GODDESS MASON JAR SALAD
LENTIL PATTIES
WHITE BEAN AND SUN-DRIED TOMATO GNOCCHI
MUSHROOM SHAWARMA WITH RICE AND GARLIC DIP
RED LENTIL PASTA WITH CREAMY TOMATO AND PEPPER SAUCE
BRAISED SESAME TOFU
GREEN GODDESS SALAD DRESSING
HARISSA BUTTER BEANS
MINI BLUEBERRY AND LEMON CHEESECAKE

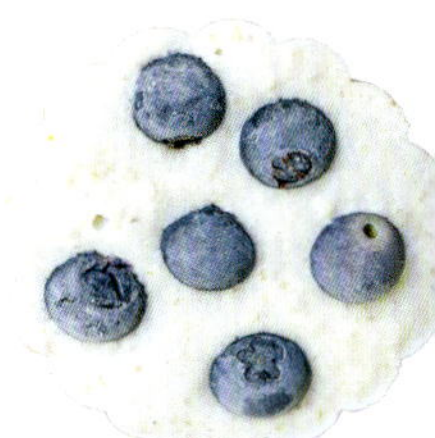

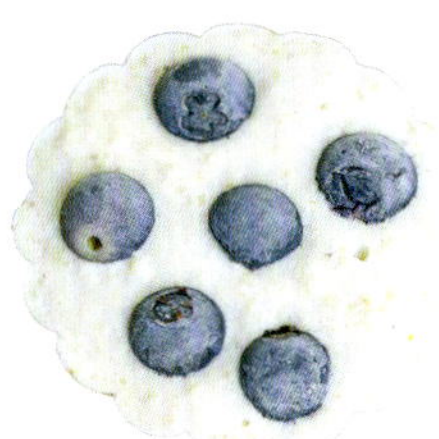

WEEKLY SHOPPING LIST

FRUITS
1 avocado
2 bananas blueberries
3 lemons
1 lime
2 oranges

VEGETABLES
2 onions
2 shallots
1 bunch green onions (spring onions)
2 bulbs garlic
root ginger
carrots
celery
cherry tomatoes
cucumber
baby spinach
rocket
button mushrooms
oyster mushrooms
broccoli
green beans

FRESH HERBS
basil chives parsley

FROZEN FOODS
edamame beans

DIRED
medjool dates
raisins
cranberries

COLD
unsweetened almond milk
oat cream (or similar plant based cream)
natural soy yogurt
14 oz (400 g) extra firm tofu

GRAINS, LEGUMES
brown rice
brown lentils (or 2 x 14 oz/ 400 g cans brown lentils)
rolled oats

NUTS, SEEDS
almonds
cashew nuts
unsweetened shredded coconut
pine nuts
hemp seeds
pumpkin seeds
sunflower seeds
sesame seeds

BAKING
all-purpose flour
self raising flour
cornstarch (corn flour)
cocoa powder

DRIED HERBS, SPICES
black pepper
smoked paprika
sweet paprika
red pepper flakes (chili flakes)
ground cinnamon
ground coriander
ground cumin
garlic powder
curry powder
garam masala
dried basil
dried oregano
dried thyme

OILS
coconut oil
olive oil

SWEETENERS
coconut
sugar
maple syrup

BOXED, CANNED, CONDIMENTS
1 x 14 oz (400 g) can cannellini beans
1 x 14 oz (400 g) can butter beans
almond butter
tahini
jar roasted red peppers
jar sun-dried tomatoes
tomato paste (purée)
harissa paste
tamari sauce
mirin
gochujang
balsamic vinegar
red wine vinegar
vegetable broth (stock)
red lentil pasta
udon noodles
gnocchi

MISC/OTHER
sea salt
nutritional yeast

Sample Weekly Meal Planner

	BREAKFAST	LUNCH
Monday	TAHINI GRANOLA	JAPANESE UDON CURRY
Tueday	VEGAN SOBRASADA (SAUSAGE SPREAD FROM MALLORCA)	RED LENTIL PASTA WITH CREAMY TOMATO AND PEPPER SAUCE
Wednesday	VEGAN SOBRASADA (SAUSAGE SPREAD FROM MALLORCA)	CARROT SOUP
Thursday	VEGAN TOMATO AND MUSHROOM PANCAKES	GREEN GODDESS MASON JAR SALAD
Friday	VEGAN TOMATO AND MUSHROOM PANCAKES	GREEN GODDESS MASON JAR SALAD
Saturday	TAHINI GRANOLA	LENTIL 'MEATBALLS'
Sunday	CHOCOLATE ALMOND DATE SMOOTHIE	JAPANESE UDON CURRY

SNACK	DINNER
E.G. CHOCOLATE ALMOND DATE SMOOTHIE, MINI BLUEBERRY AND LEMON CHEESECAKE, HARISSA, BUTTER BEANS	RED LENTIL PASTA WITH CREAMY TOMATO AND PEPPER SAUCE
E.G. CHOCOLATE ALMOND DATE SMOOTHIE, MINI BLUEBERRY AND LEMON CHEESECAKE, HARISSA, BUTTER BEANS	WHITE BEAN AND SUN-DRIED TOMATO GNOCCHI
E.G. CHOCOLATE ALMOND DATE SMOOTHIE, MINI BLUEBERRY AND LEMON CHEESECAKE, HARISSA, BUTTER BEANS	MUSHROOM SHAWARMA WITH RICE AND GARLIC DIP
E.G. CHOCOLATE ALMOND DATE SMOOTHIE, MINI BLUEBERRY AND LEMON CHEESECAKE, HARISSA, BUTTER BEANS	MUSHROOM SHAWARMA WITH RICE AND GARLIC DIP
E.G. CHOCOLATE ALMOND DATE SMOOTHIE, MINI BLUEBERRY AND LEMON CHEESECAKE, HARISSA, BUTTER BEANS	LENTIL 'MEATBALLS'
E.G. CHOCOLATE ALMOND DATE SMOOTHIE, MINI BLUEBERRY AND LEMON CHEESECAKE, HARISSA, BUTTER BEANS	MEAL OUT – ENJOY!
E.G. CHOCOLATE ALMOND DATE SMOOTHIE, MINI BLUEBERRY AND LEMON CHEESECAKE, HARISSA, BUTTER BEANS	BRAISED SESAME TOFU

SERVES **2** | **5** MINUTES

CHOCOLATE ALMOND DATE SMOOTHIE

INGREDIENTS

8 fl oz (240 ml) **unsweetened almond milk**
2 **bananas**, frozen
2 tbsp **cocoa powder**, unsweetened
1 tbsp **almond butter**
2 **medjool dates**

METHOD

- Place all the ingredients into a high-speed blender and blend until smooth. Divide the smoothie equally between 2 glasses and serve.
- Storage: Best enjoyed immediately, but can be stored in the refrigerator. Consume within 24 hours for the best taste.

ENERGY: **283** kcal	CARBS: **50** g	PROTEIN: **5** g	FAT: **7** g	FIBRE: **6** g

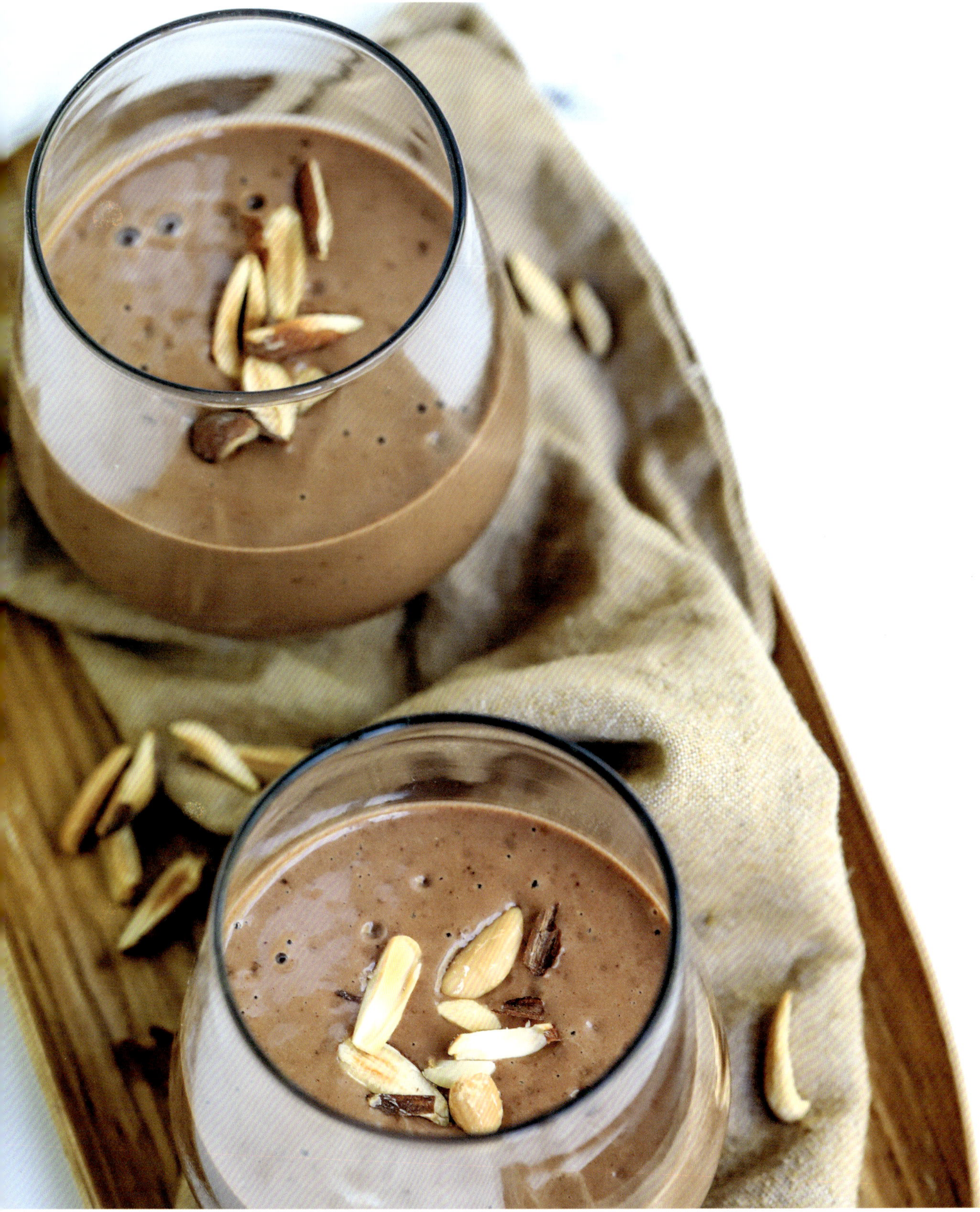

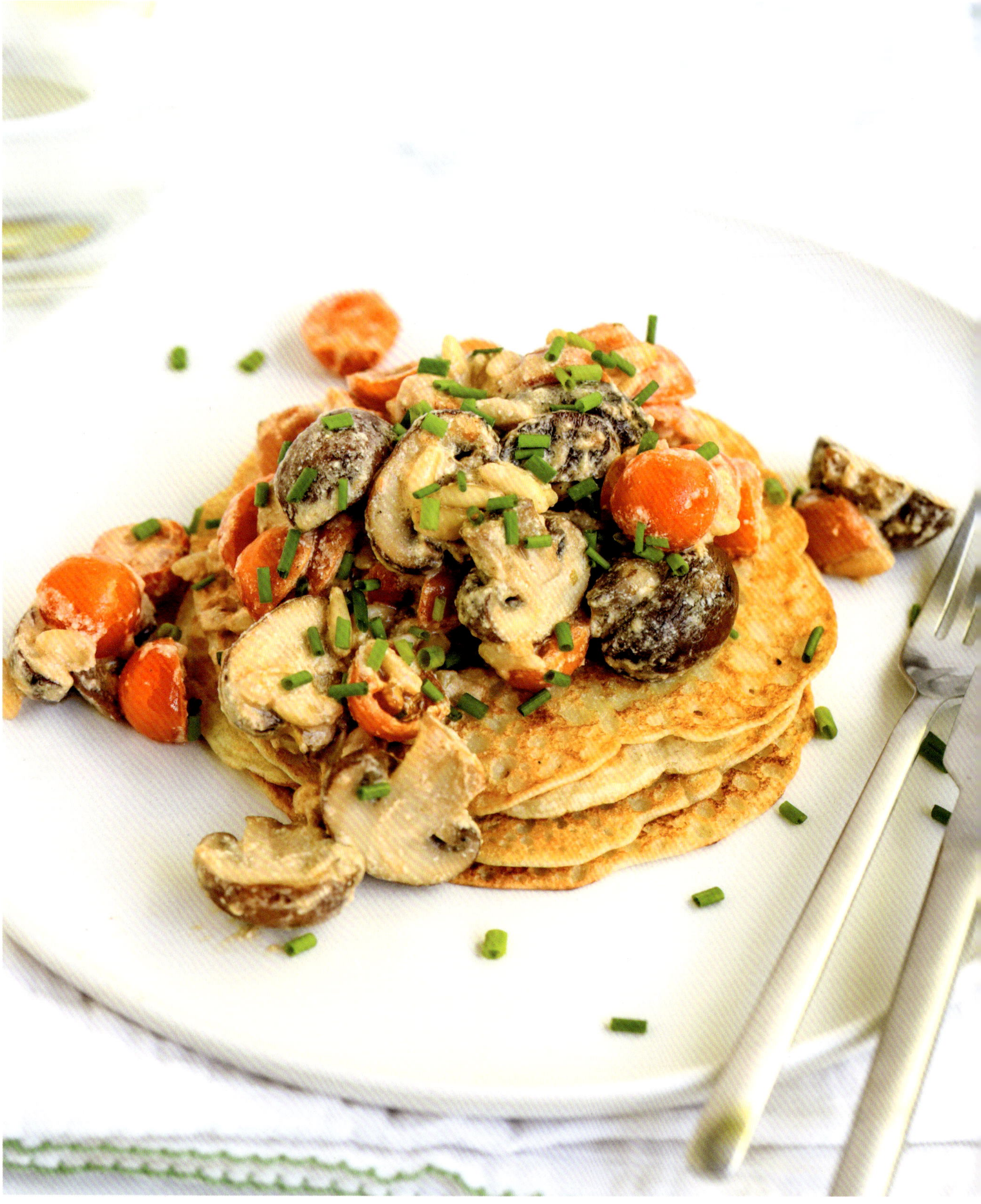

SERVES **2** | **30** MINUTES

VEGAN TOMATO AND MUSHROOM **PANCAKES**

INGREDIENTS

5 oz (140 g) **self-raising flour**
pinch of **sea salt**
13.5 fl oz (400 ml) **unsweetened almond milk**
1 tbsp **olive oil**

For the topping

1 tbsp **olive oil**
8.8 oz (250 g) **button mushrooms**
8.8 oz (250 g) **cherry tomatoes**, halved
2 tbsp **oat cream**
2 tbsp **pine nuts**
2 tbsp **chives**, chopped, to serve

METHOD

- Sift the flour and salt into a blender. Add the milk and blend until smooth to make a pancake batter.
- Heat a little of the olive oil in a non-stick skillet over medium heat until very hot. Pour about 3 tablespoons of the batter into the skillet. Cook until bubbles appear on the surface of the pancake, then flip it over and cook the other side until golden brown. Remove the pancake from the skillet and set aside to keep warm. Repeat this process with the remaining olive oil and pancake batter.
- To make the topping, heat the olive oil in a skillet, add the mushrooms and cook until tender. Now add the tomatoes and cook for a further 2–3 minutes. Pour in the oat cream and add the pine nuts, cooking gently until everything is well combined.
- To serve, divide the pancakes between 2 plates, spoon the mushroom and tomato mixture over the pancakes, and garnish with chives.
- **Storage:** These pancakes are best served fresh but can be stored in the refrigerator for up to 2 days and reheated before serving.

ENERGY: **469** kcal | CARBS: **68** g | PROTEIN: **11** g | FAT: **17** g

SERVES **4** | **5** MINUTES

VEGAN SOBRASADA

INGREDIENTS

5.3 oz (150 g) **sun-dried tomatoes,** drained
2 oz (60 g) **raw cashews**
1 clove **garlic**
2 tbsp **olive oil**
1½ tbsp **sweet paprika**
1 tsp **dried basil**
½ tsp **ground cumin**
pinch of **salt**
4 tbsp **water**

METHOD

- Place all the ingredients into a blender and blitz to a paste.
- Store the mixture in a sealed jar in the refrigerator. Serve on top of bread or with vegetables.

ENERGY: **271** kcal | CARBS: **26** g | PROTEIN: **8** g | FAT: **15** g

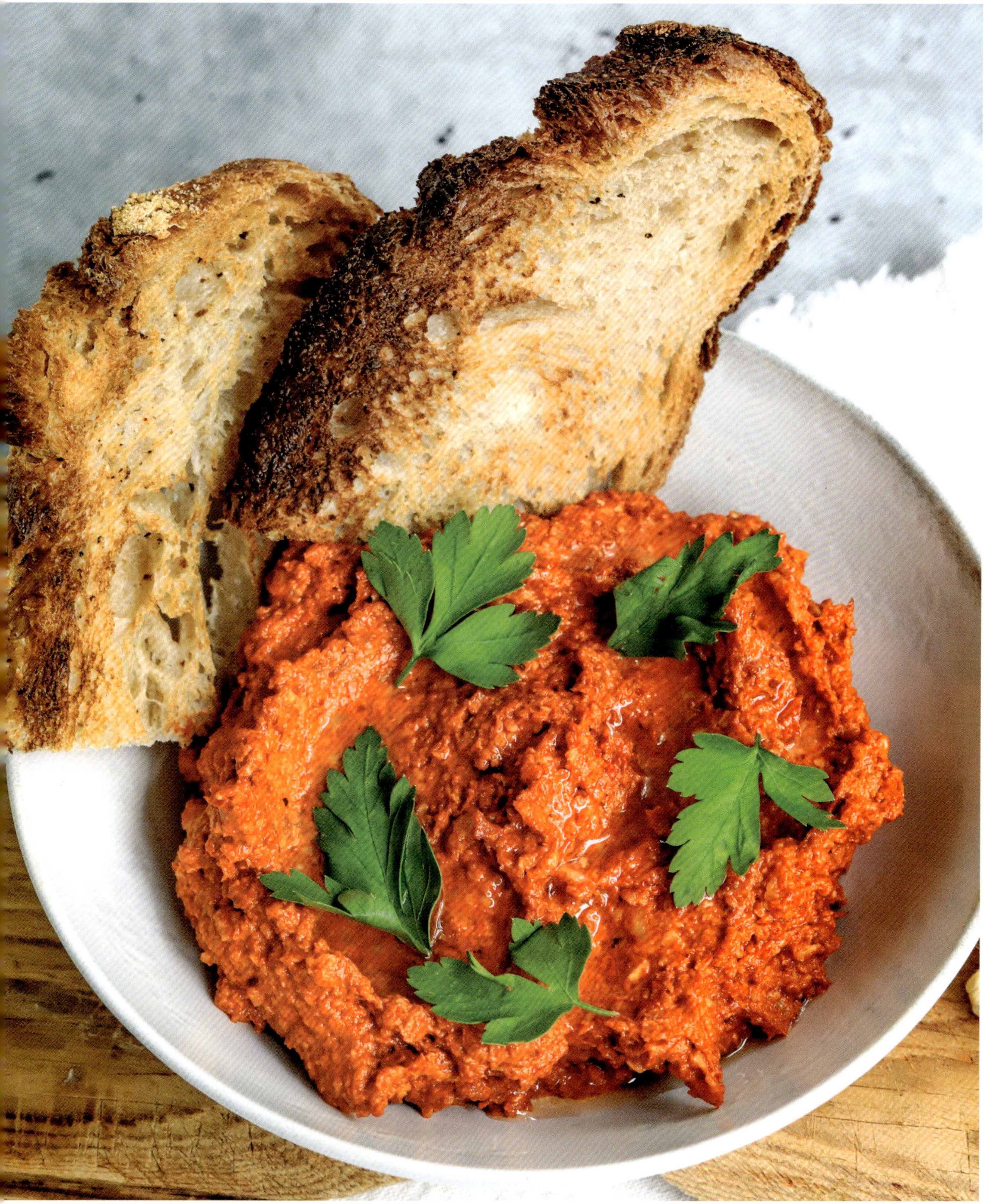

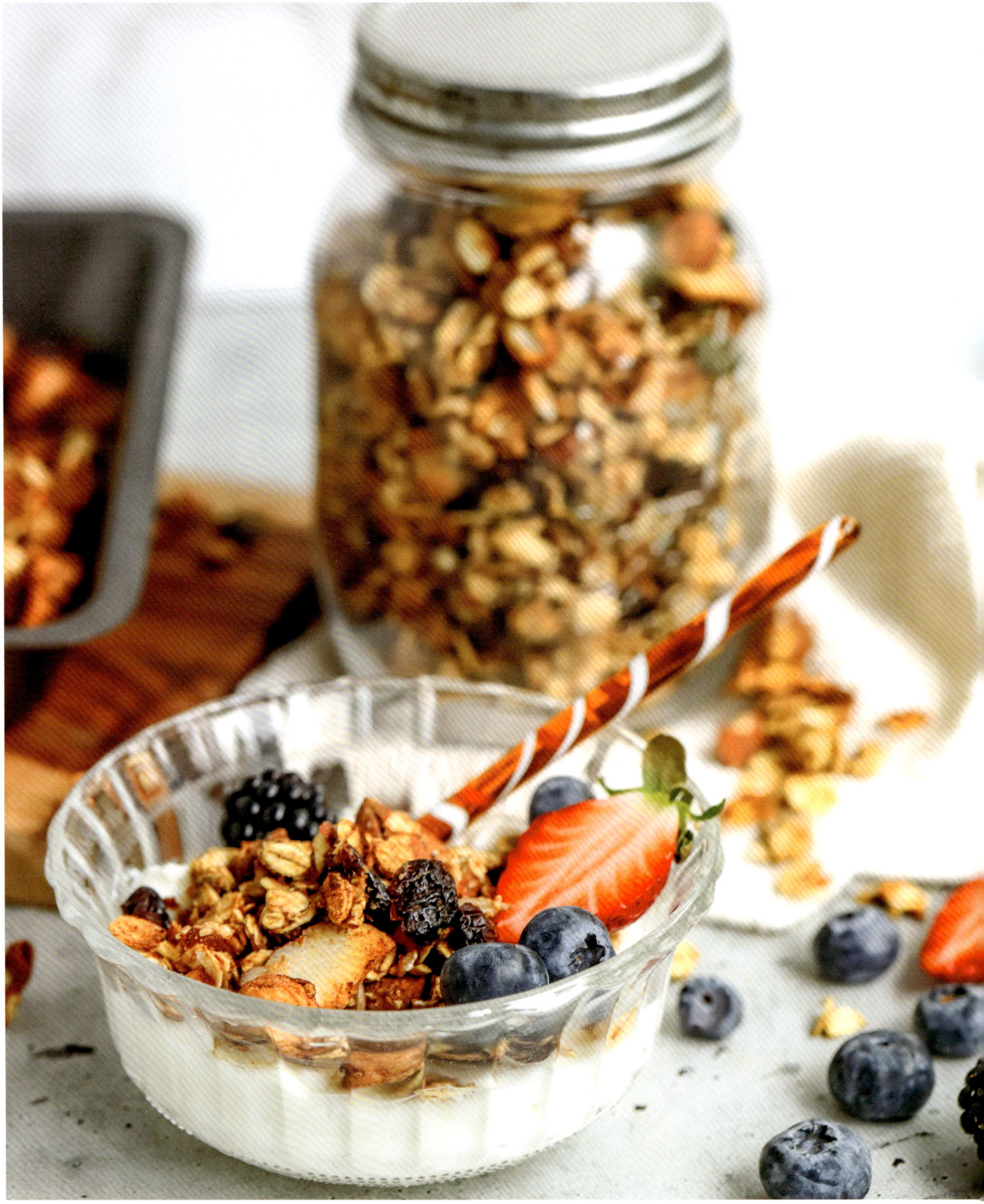

SERVES **13** | **30** MINUTES

TAHINI GRANOLA

INGREDIENTS

6 oz (170 g) **medjool dates**, pitted
4 fl oz (120 ml) **tahini**
1.5 fl oz (45 ml) **water**
10.6 oz (300 g) **rolled oats**
2.8 oz (80 g) **raw almonds**, roughly chopped
2.3 oz (65 g) **raw cashews**, roughly chopped
2.8 oz (80 g) **raisins**
1.4 oz (40 g) **dried cranberries**
1.4 oz (40 g) **sunflower seeds**
1.4 oz (40 g) **pumpkin seeds**
0.7 oz (20 g) **unsweetened shredded coconut**
½ tsp **ground cinnamon**
¼ tsp **sea salt**

METHOD

- Preheat the oven to 300°F (150°C). Line a baking tray with parchment paper.
- In a small food processor, combine the dates, tahini and water. Blend on high until the mixture is creamy.
- Place the remaining ingredients into a large bowl and stir until well combined.
- Pour the date mixture into the bowl with the dry ingredients. Mix thoroughly to ensure all ingredients are evenly coated. Then spread the granola mixture evenly on the prepared baking tray.
- Place the baking tray into the centre rack of the oven and bake for 25–30 minutes, stirring once or twice during baking to prevent burning and to promote an even cook.
- Once the granola is lightly golden, remove the tray from the oven and set aside on a wire rack to cool.
- Once completely cooled, transfer the granola to an airtight container or a large glass storage jar.

Serving suggestion: Enjoy this granola with your choice of milk or yogurt; or as a crunchy topping for smoothie bowls.
Storage: For optimal freshness, store the granola in a sealed container on the countertop for up to 2 weeks.

ENERGY: **273** Kcal | CARBS: **32** g | PROTEIN: **7** g | FATS: **13** g

JAPANESE CURRY **UDON**

INGREDIENTS

For the vegetables

1 tbsp **olive oil**
1 tbsp **ginger**, minced
1 **clove garlic**, minced
½ yellow **onion**, sliced into thin strips
1 **stalk celery**, diced small

For the curry

3 tbsp **olive oil**
3 tbsp **flour**
1 tbsp + 1 tsp **curry powder**
1 tsp **garam masala**
½ tsp **sea salt**
1 pint (480 ml) **vegetable broth**
14 oz (400 g) **fresh udon noodles**

METHOD

- 2 green onions, sliced, for garnish.
- Place a pot over medium heat and warm up the olive oil. Add the ginger and garlic, and sauté for 1 minute.
- Add the onions and sauté for an additional minute, then add the celery and continue to sauté until all the vegetables are tender, approximately 3 minutes. Remove the vegetables from the pot and set aside.
- Now make the curry sauce in the same pot. Add the olive oil and once melted whisk in the flour, curry powder, garam masala and salt. Cook for 1 minute to bloom the spices and cook the flour.
- Gradually add the vegetable broth a little at a time, whisking continuously to ensure the sauce is smooth and free of lumps before adding more stock. Once all the stock has been added, increase the heat to medium-high and continue whisking until the sauce thickens and starts to bubble, approximately 1–2 minutes.
- Return the cooked veggies to the pot and reduce the heat to low.
- Bring a separate pot of salted water to a boil. Add the udon noodles and cook for 1 minute less than the package instructions suggest. Drain the noodles.
- Add the drained noodles to the pot with the curry sauce. Mix well to coat the noodles in the sauce and cook together for an additional minute.
- Garnish the noodles with sliced green onions and serve immediately.
- Storage: Store leftovers in an airtight container in the refrigerator for up to 3 days and reheat gently on the stove or in the microwave.

ENERGY: **438** Kcal	CARBS: **82** g	PROTEIN: **14** g	Fats **6** g

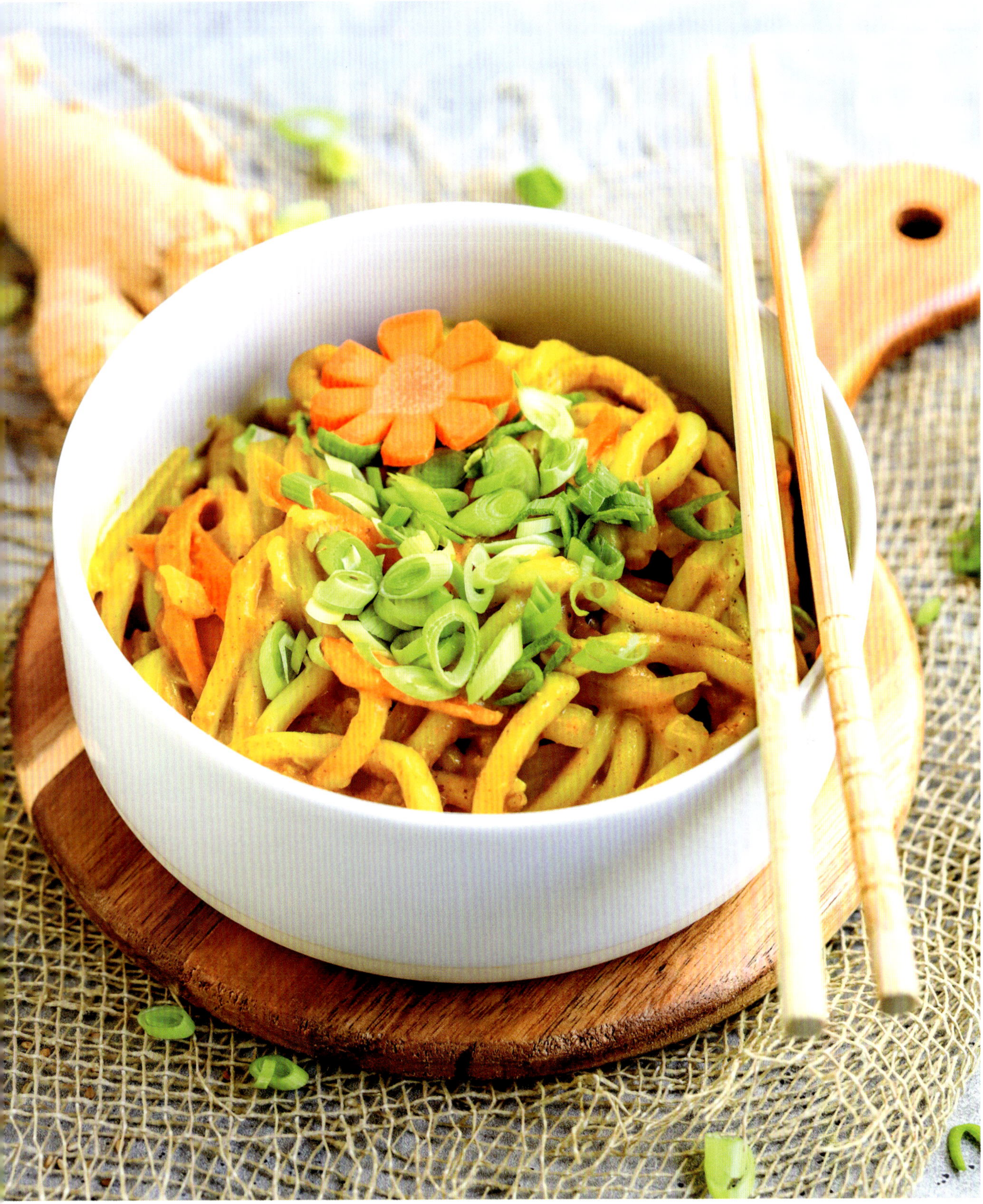

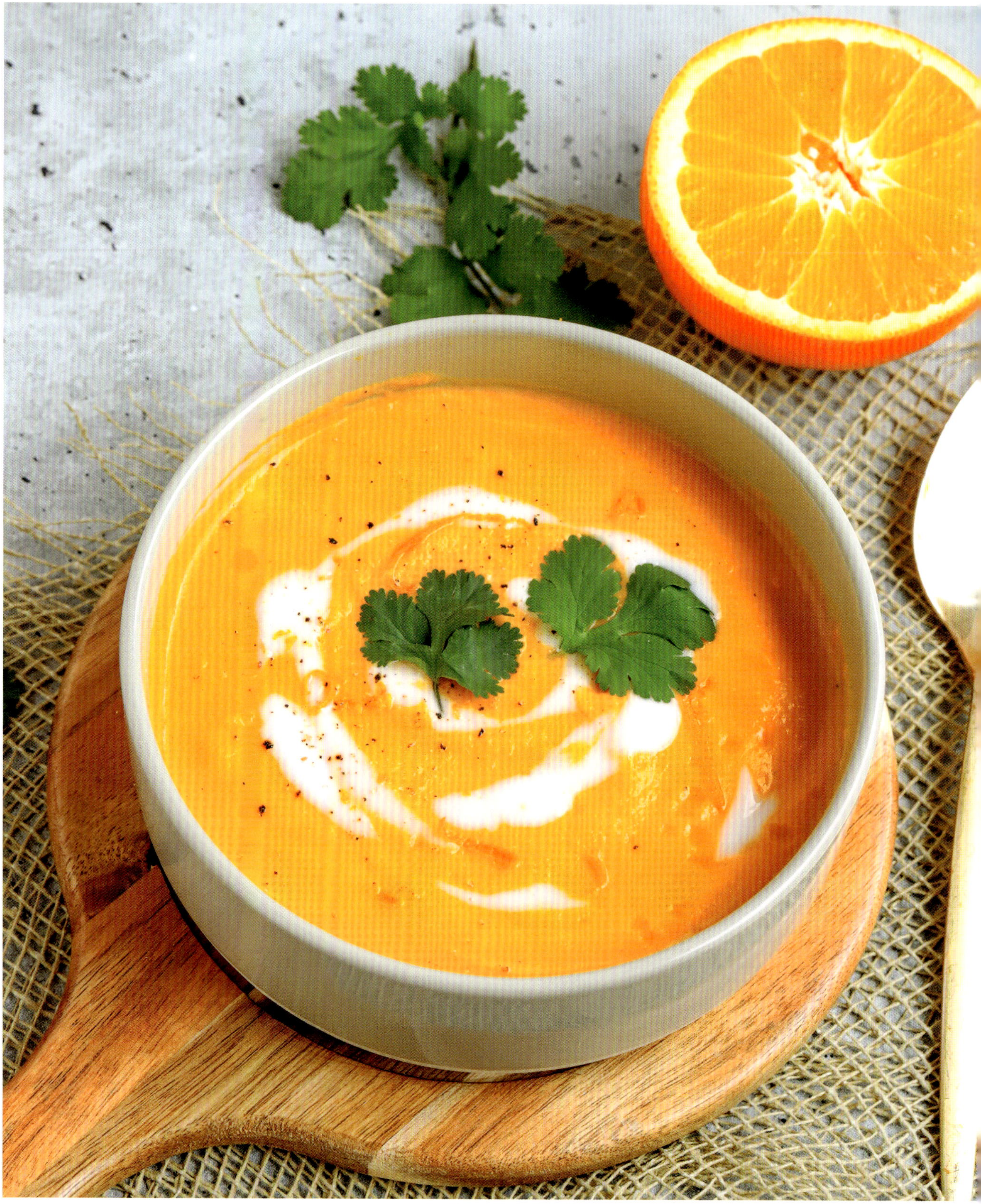

SERVES **2** | **20** MINUTES

CARROT SOUP

INGREDIENTS

1 tbsp **olive oil**
1 **shallot**, finely chopped
10.6 oz (300 g) **carrots**, cut into pieces
½ tsp **ground coriander**
sea salt, to taste
black pepper, to taste
zest and juice of 2 **oranges**
500 ml **vegetable broth**
1 tsp **coconut sugar**
1 tbsp **oat cream**

METHOD

- Place a medium pot over medium heat, add the olive oil. Now add the shallot and sauté for 2–3 minutes until translucent.
- Add the carrots to the pot stirring to combine with the shallots. Cook for an additional 5 minutes, until the carrots start to soften slightly. Season with ground coriander, salt and pepper and stir to combine.
- Stir in the orange zest, orange juice and vegetable broth. Bring the mixture to a simmer, then cover and cook for approximately 25 minutes, or until the carrots are very soft.
- Remove from heat. Using an immersion blender, purée the soup in the pot until smooth.
- Alternatively, carefully transfer the soup to a blender and purée.
- Now stir in the sugar and adjust the seasoning to taste with a little more salt and pepper. Ladle the soup into warmed soup bowls and top each bowl with a little oat cream.

ENERGY: **209** kcal	CARBS: **29** g	PROTEIN: **9** g	Fats **3** g

GREEN GODDESS MASON JAR SALAD

INGREDIENTS

1.6 oz (45 g) **dry brown rice**

2 servings **Green Goddess Salad Dressing** (see recipe on p 150)

5.3 oz (150 g) **frozen edamame**, thawed

0.7 oz (20 g) **broccoli**, cut into florets

½ **cucumber**, diced

2 oz (60 g) **baby spinach**

2 tbsp **hemp seeds**

METHOD

- Cook the rice according to the package directions. Once cooked, drain and set aside to cool to room temperature.
- Assemble the salad in a 16 fl oz (475 ml) mason jar in the following order to ensure optimal freshness.
- Pour the Green Goddess Salad Dressing into the base of the jar. Add the thawed edamame, followed by the broccoli florets and then the cooled brown rice. Top the rice with the diced cucumber, then the baby spinach and finish with the hemp seeds on top.
- Seal the jar tightly with the lid and refrigerate until ready to serve.
- When ready to eat, shake the jar well to distribute the dressing evenly throughout the salad. Divide the contents equally between 2 bowls and serve.
- Storage: The sealed mason jar salad can be stored in the refrigerator for up to 3 days.

ENERGY: **353** kcal	CARBS: **34** g	PROTEIN: **16** g	FAT: **17** g

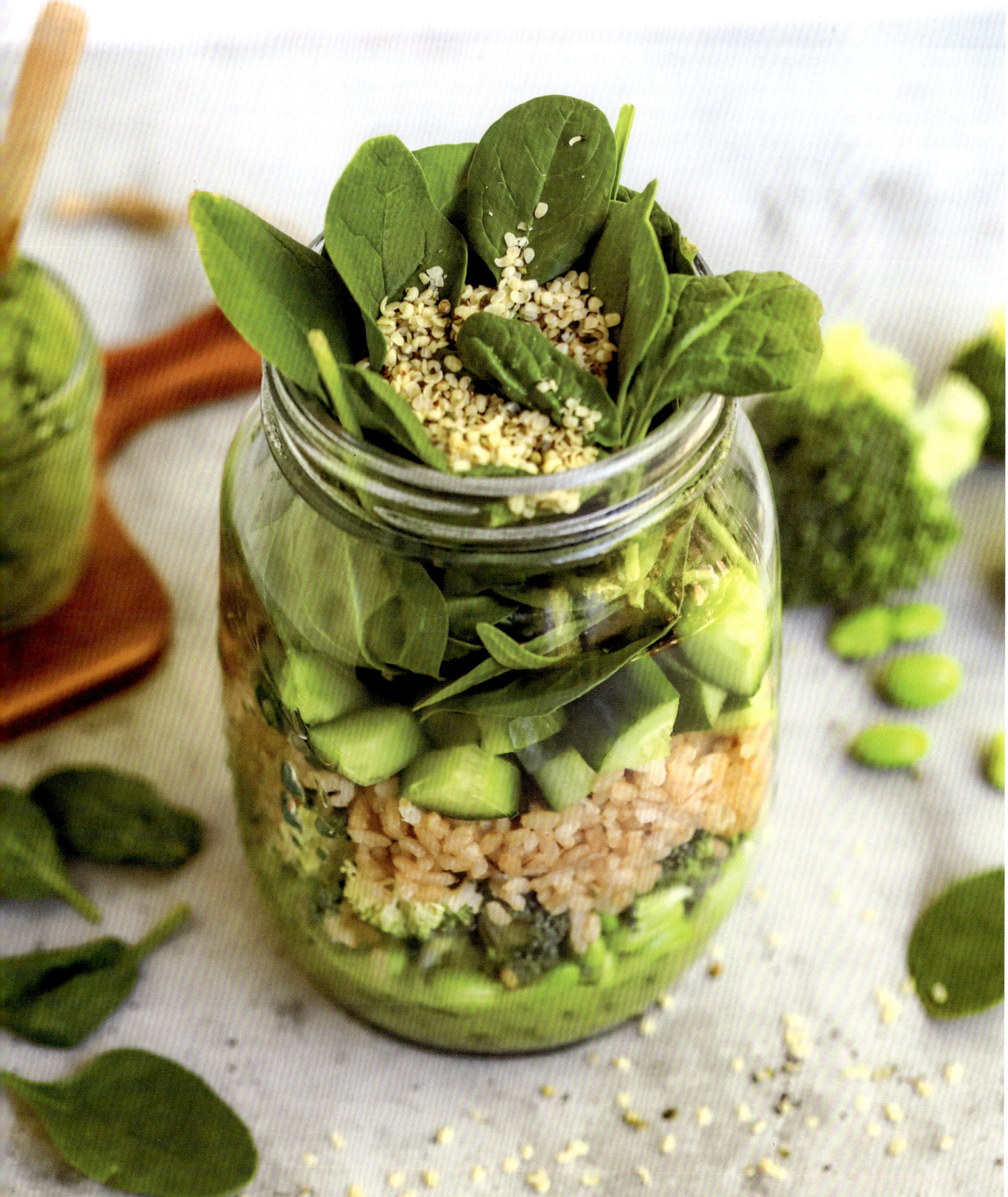

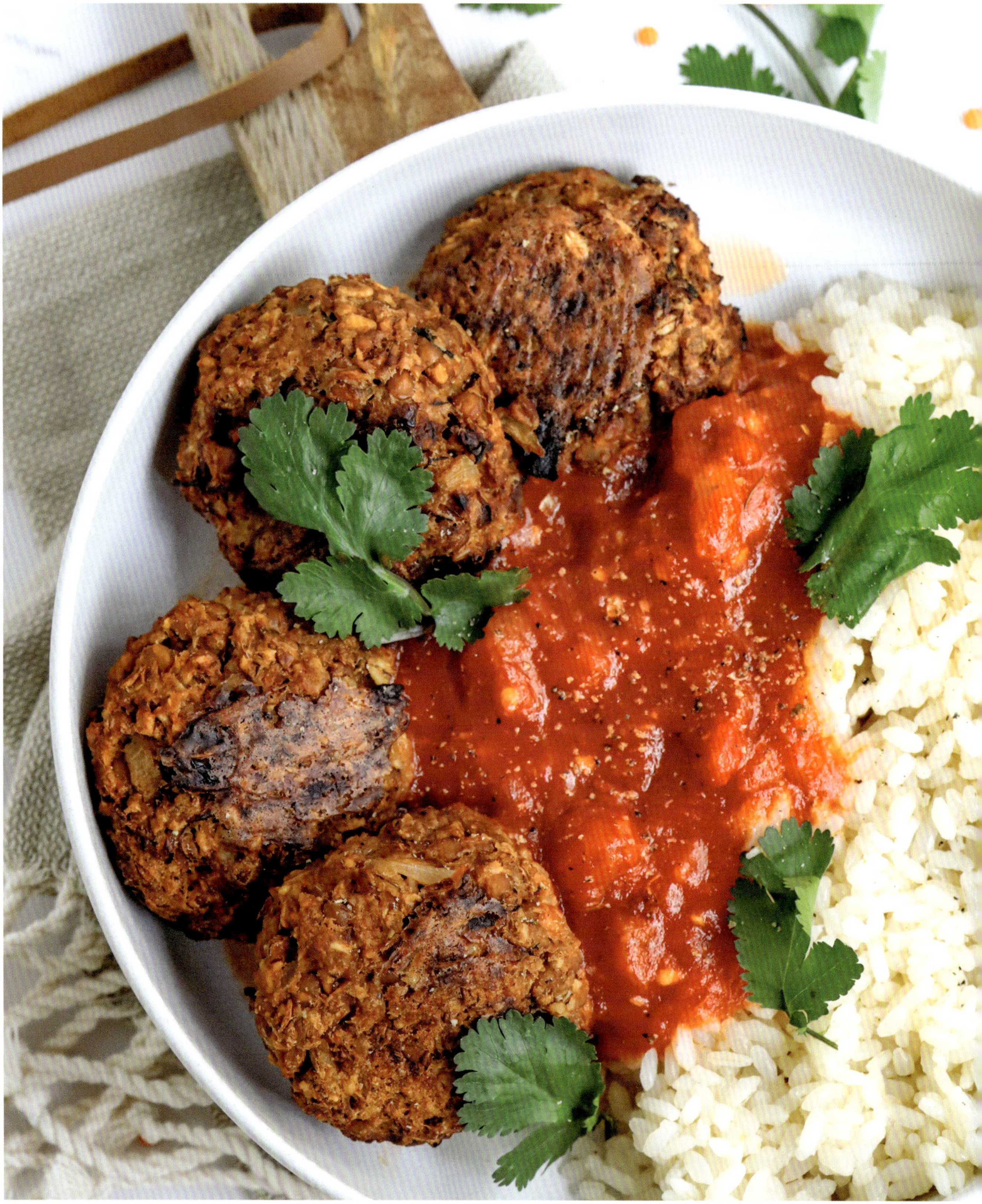

SERVES **4** | **40** MINUTES

LENTIL **PATTIES**

INGREDIENTS

2 tbsp **olive oil**, divided
1 **onion**, diced
3 cloves **garlic**, minced (divided)
2.8 oz (80 g) **rolled oats**
14 oz (400 g) **cooked** or **canned brown lentils**
2 tbsp **tomato paste**
1 tbsp **tamari sauce**
1½ tsp **red wine vinegar**
1 tsp **dried oregano**
1 tsp **dried thyme**
1 tsp **dried basil**
½ tsp **red pepper** flakes, or to taste
½ tsp **sea salt**, or to taste
½ tsp **black pepper**, or to taste

METHOD

- Preheat the oven to 400°F (200°C). Lightly oil a baking sheet or an oven-safe skillet.
- Heat 1 tablespoon of olive oil in a medium skillet over medium heat. Add the onion and sauté for 5 minutes until soft and translucent. Add 2 cloves of minced garlic and continue sautéing for another minute until fragrant. Remove from heat.
- Place the rolled oats in a food processor and process until they reach a powdery consistency. Add the remaining clove of garlic, cooked lentils, tomato paste, tamari sauce, red wine vinegar, oregano, thyme, basil, red pepper flakes, salt and black pepper to the food processor, pulse a few times until combined but still retaining some texture. Be careful not to over-process the mixture, it should not be smooth.
- Taste the mixture and adjust the seasoning if needed. Now roll the mixture into walnut-sized patties (this mixture should make around 24 patties).
- Arrange the balls on the prepared baking sheet and brush or spray them with the remaining tablespoon of olive oil. Place in the hot oven to bake for about 24 minutes, flipping halfway through, until the balls are firm and lightly browned.
- Serve the lentil patties with your favourite sauce.
- Storage: Store leftovers in an airtight container in the refrigerator for up to 5 days. Reheat in the oven or microwave.
- Freezing: Store uncooked or cooked lentil meatballs in the freezer for up to 3 months. Thaw in the refrigerator overnight before cooking or reheating.

ENERGY: **228** kcal | CARBS: **30** g | PROTEIN: **9** g | FAT: **9** g | FIBRE: **8** g

SERVES **4** | **15** MINUTES

WHITE BEAN AND SUN-DRIED TOMATO GNOCCHI

INGREDIENTS

1 lb (450 g) **gnocchi**
1 x 14 oz can **cannellini beans**, rinsed
5 oz (140 g) **baby spinach**
3.5 oz (100 g) **sun-dried tomatoes**, drained, sliced + 1 tbsp oil from the jar
1 **shallot**, minced
2.7 fl oz (80 ml) **vegetable broth**
2.7 fl oz (80 ml) **oat cream**
1 tbsp **lemon juice**
¼ tsp **sea salt**
¼ tsp **black pepper**
3 tbsp **fresh basil leaves**, for garnish

METHOD

- Cook the gnocchi according to the package instructions. Drain the gnocchi and add to a skillet, along with the cannellini beans and spinach. Cook gently over medium heat until the spinach has wilted then remove from the skillet and set aside on a plate.
- Add a tablespoon of sun-dried tomato oil to the skillet and place over medium heat. Add the sun-dried tomatoes and shallot, and cook, stirring frequently, for 1 minute.
- Increase the heat to high and add the broth to the skillet. Cook for approximately 2 minutes until the liquid has almost evaporated.
- Reduce the heat to medium and stir in the oat cream, lemon juice, salt and pepper.
- Return the gnocchi mixture to the skillet. Stir well to ensure the gnocchi and vegetables are coated with the sauce. Heat through until everything is warm, about 1–2 minutes.
- Spoon the gnocchi into bowls or onto plates. Garnish with fresh basil leaves and serve immediately. Storage: Store leftovers in an airtight container in the refrigerator for up to 2 days. Reheat gently in the microwave or on the stovetop.

ENERGY: **376** kcal | CARBS: **65** g | PROTEIN: **12** g | FAT: **8** g | FIBRE: **8** g

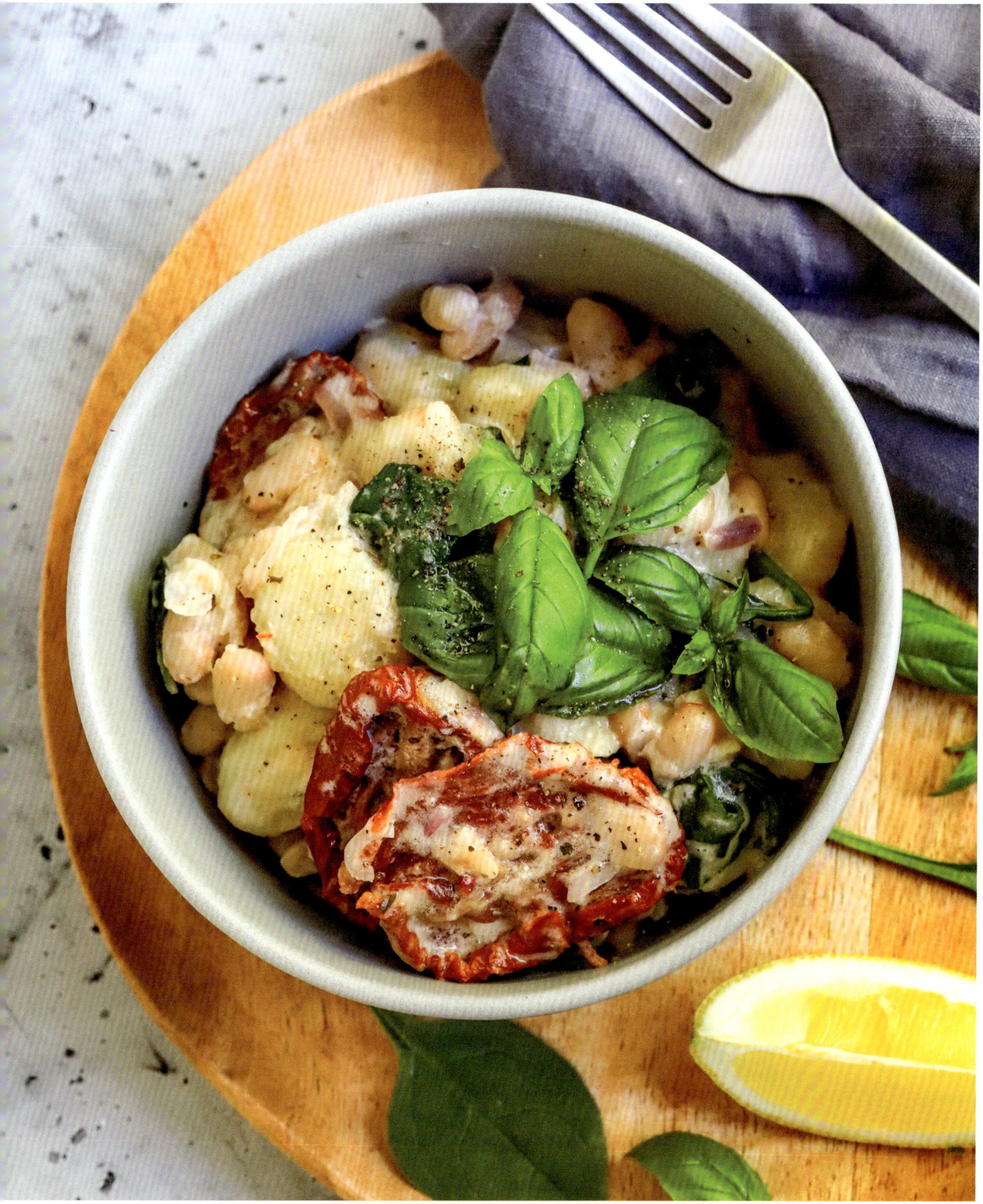

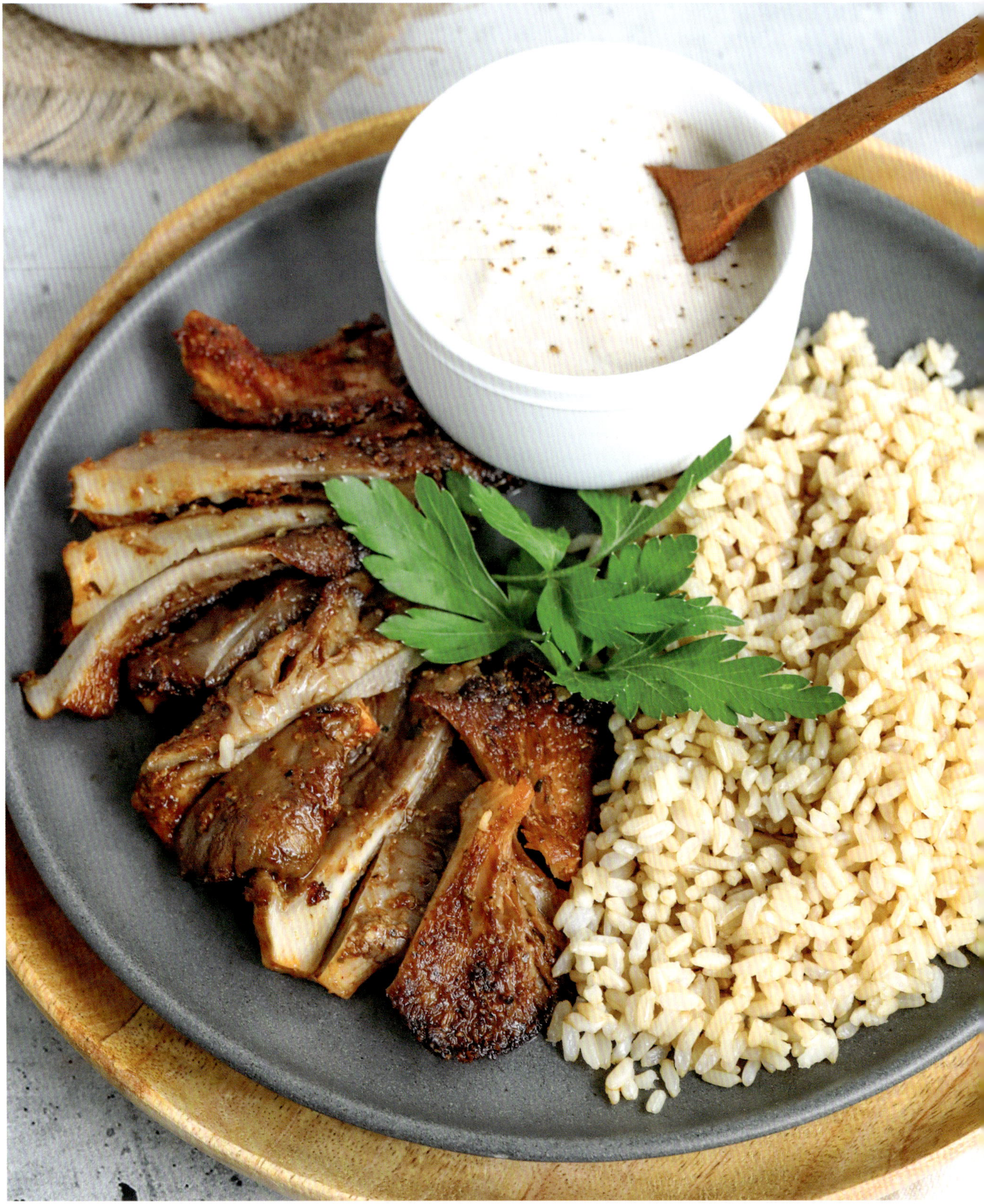

SERVES **4** | **20** MINUTES

MUSHROOM SHAWARMA WITH RICE AND GARLIC DIP

INGREDIENTS

For the shawarma

1 lb (450 g) **oyster mushrooms**
3 tbsp **olive oil**
1 tsp **ground cumin**
2 tsp **dried oregano**
2 tsp **smoked paprika**
2 tbsp **nutritional yeast**
3 tsp **cornstarch**
1 tsp **salt**
1 tsp **garlic powder**

For the garlic yogurt

7 oz (200 g) **natural soy yogurt**
juice of one **lemon**
2 cloves **garlic**, minced
1 tbsp **balsamic vinegar**
2 tsp **maple syrup**
sea salt and **black pepper**, to taste
1 lb (480 g) **cooked brown rice**, to serve

METHOD

- In a large bowl, combine the oyster mushrooms with 1 tablespoon of the olive oil and remaining shawarma ingredients. Toss until mushrooms are evenly coated.
- Heat the remaining 2 tablespoons of olive oil in a skillet, over medium-high heat. Add the seasoned mushrooms and sauté for 5–7 minutes until lightly browned. Transfer the mushrooms to a plate and, once cool enough to handle, cut them into strips.
- Place all the ingredients for the garlic yogurt into a bowl and season to taste with salt and pepper.
- Serve the mushroom shawarma strips, alongside the cooked brown rice and garlic yogurt.
- Storage: Store leftovers separately in airtight containers. The shawarma can be refrigerated for up to 3 days. The garlic yogurt should be consumed within 1–2 days for best flavour.

ENERGY: **312** kcal	CARBS: **41** g	PROTEIN: **10** g	FAT: **4** g	FIBRE: **4** g

SERVES **2** | **18** MINUTES

RED LENTIL PASTA WITH CREAMY TOMATO AND PEPPER SAUCE

INGREDIENTS

large pinch of **salt**
5.3 oz (150 g) **red lentil pasta**
1 oz (30 g) **rocket**

For the sauce

2 oz (60 g) **cashews**
1 **clove garlic**, roughly chopped
4.2 fl oz (125 ml) **boiling water**
1 **large roasted red pepper**, from a jar, drained
4 **sun-dried tomatoes**
8 **large basil leaves**, roughly chopped
black pepper, to taste

METHOD

- Place the cashews and chopped garlic in a bowl. Pour over the boiling water and set aside for 5 minutes to soften the cashews.
- Add the roasted red pepper and sun-dried tomatoes to the bowl with the cashews and garlic. Use a hand blender or transfer to a food processor to blend until smooth.
- Stir the chopped basil into the sauce and season with black pepper to taste.
- Bring a large pot of water to a rapid boil. Add a pinch of salt to the pot, then the fusilli. Stir once, then boil for 8 minutes, or according to the package instructions, until the pasta is al dente.
- Drain the pasta and transfer it to a large bowl. Pour the prepared sauce over the pasta and mix well to combine.
- Divide the pasta between 2 bowls and top each with a handful of rocket.
- Storage: Leftovers can be stored in an airtight container in the refrigerator for up to 2 days.

ENERGY: **423** kcal	CARBS: **53** g	PROTEIN: **19** g	FAT: **15** g	FIBRE: **7** g

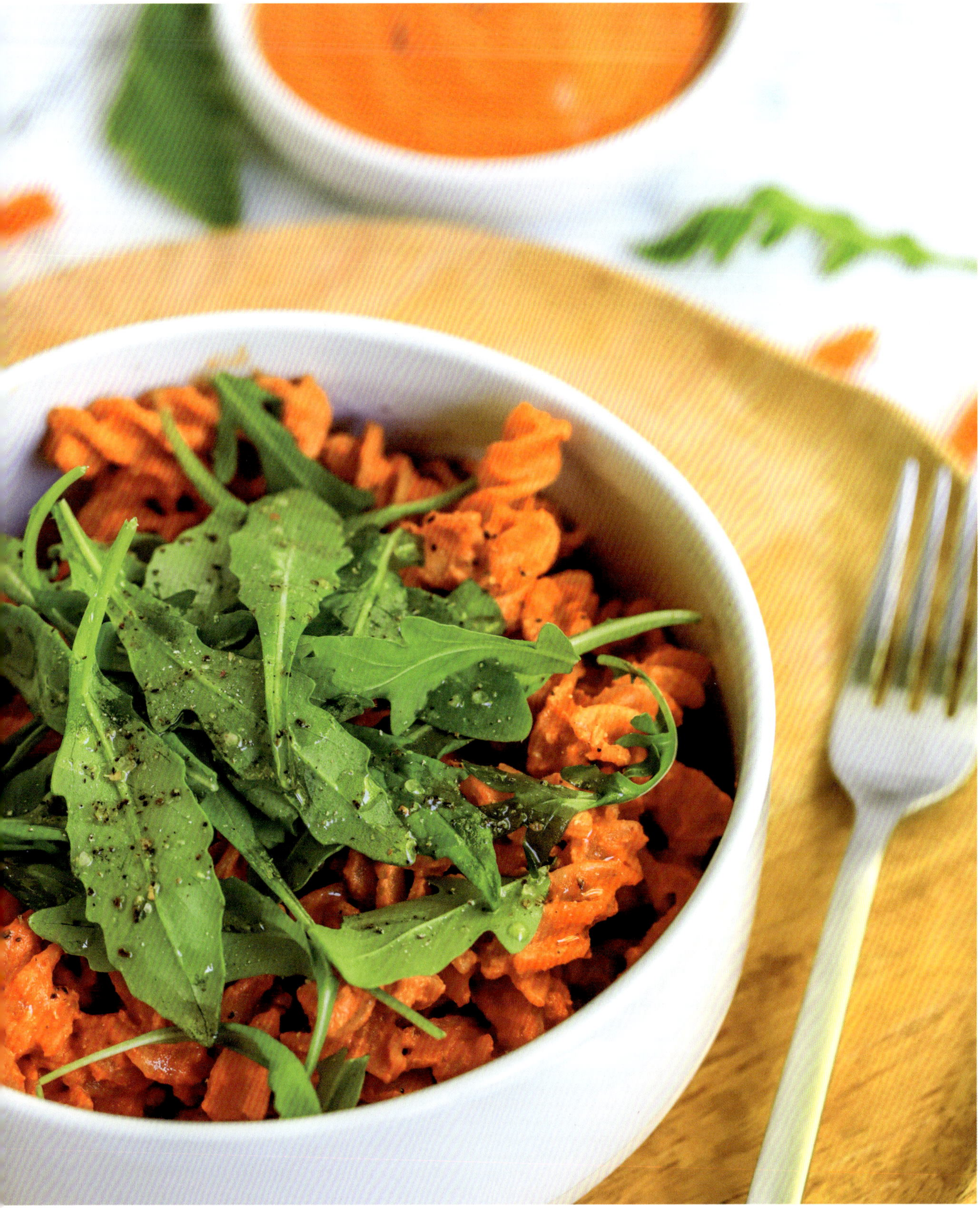

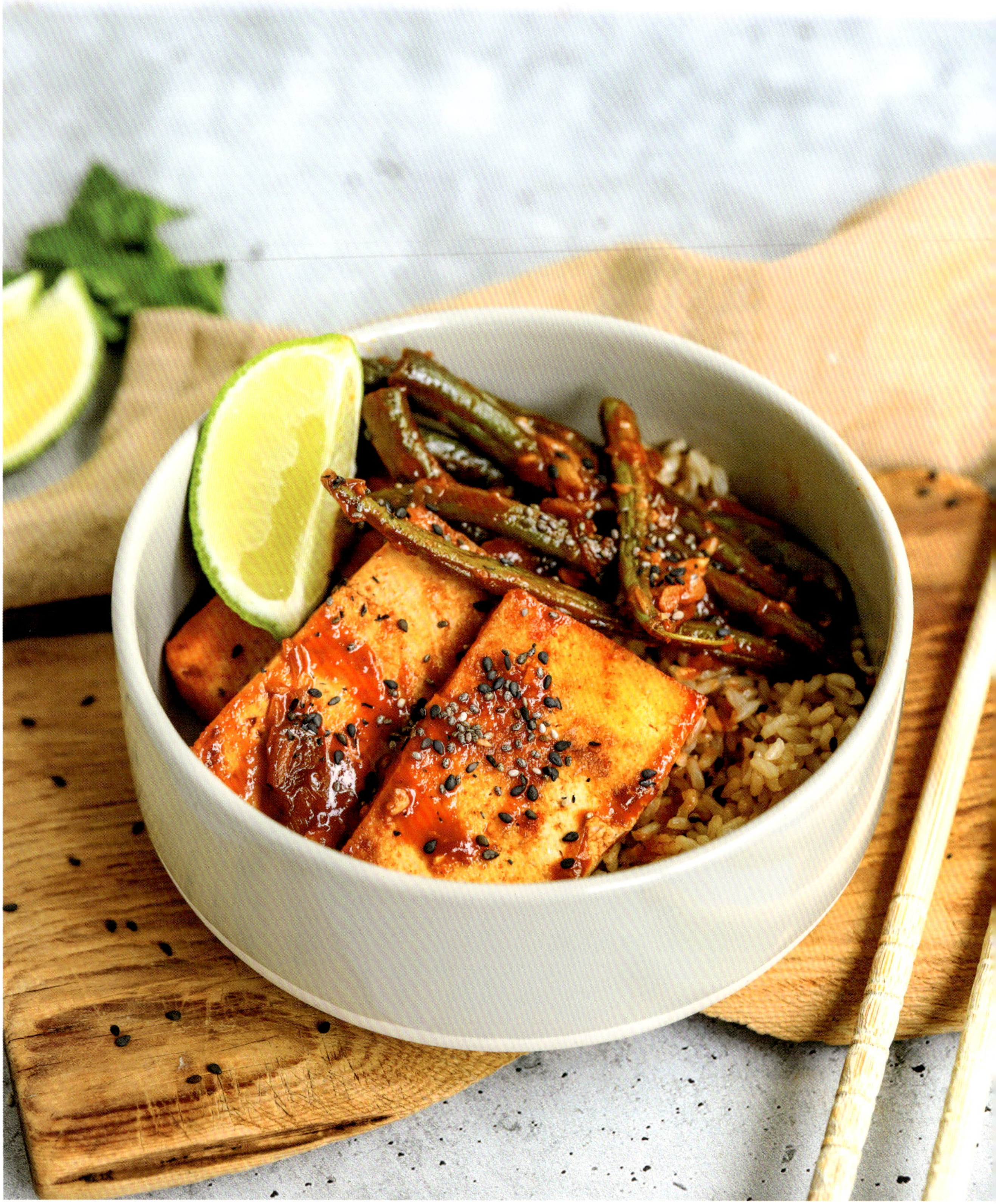

SERVES **2** | **25** MINUTES

BRAISED SESAME **TOFU**

INGREDIENTS

14 oz (400 g) **extra-firm tofu**
½ tbsp **tamari**
1 tbsp **mirin**
½ tbsp **gochujang**
3 cloves **garlic**, finely chopped
2 tsp **sesame seeds**
2 **green onions**, finely sliced, divided
6.8 fl oz (200 ml) **water**
1 tbsp **coconut oil**
7 oz (200 g) **green beans**
1 **lime**, juiced
sea salt, to taste
15 oz (440 g) **cooked brown rice**, for serving

METHOD

- Pat the tofu dry with kitchen paper. Cut it in half lengthways, then slice into 1 cm thick pieces. Arrange the slices on a plate lined with kitchen paper. Cover with another sheet of paper and place a second plate on top to weigh it down. Set aside to drain.
- In a small bowl, add the tamari, mirin, gochujang, garlic, sesame seeds, most of the green onions (reserving some for garnish) and water, and stir to combine.
- Heat the coconut oil in a non-stick skillet over medium-high heat. Add the tofu slices and sauté for 4–5 minutes on each side, or until golden brown.
- Pour the sauce mixture over the sautéed tofu in the skillet. Scatter the green beans around the tofu. Bring the mixture to a simmer and cook for 10 minutes over medium heat, or until the sauce has thickened and the green beans are tender.
- Sprinkle the reserved green onions over the dish. Squeeze lime juice over the top to taste and season with additional salt if needed. Serve hot alongside the cooked brown rice.
- Storage: Leftovers can be stored in an airtight container in the refrigerator for up to 3 days. Reheat gently before serving.

ENERGY: **581** kcal | CARBS: **69** g | PROTEIN: **29** g | FAT: **21** g | FIBRE: **6** g

SERVES **4** | **10** MINUTES

GREEN GODDESS SALAD DRESSING

INGREDIENTS

1 **avocado**
1 oz (30 g) **parsley**, stems removed
1 **green onion**, trimmed and chopped
sea salt, to taste
8 fl oz (240 ml) **water**, divided

METHOD

- In a food processor, add the avocado, parsley, green onion, sea salt and approximately half of the water (about 4 fl oz/120 ml).
- Process until smooth. Pause to scrape down the sides of the food processor as needed to ensure everything is well blended.
- Gradually add more water, one tablespoon at a time, to achieve the desired consistency.
- Enjoy immediately, or store for later use.
- Storage: Store the sauce in an airtight container in the refrigerator for up to 3 days.

ENERGY: **87** kcal	CARBS: **5** g	PROTEIN: **1** g	FAT: **7** g	FIBRE: **4** g

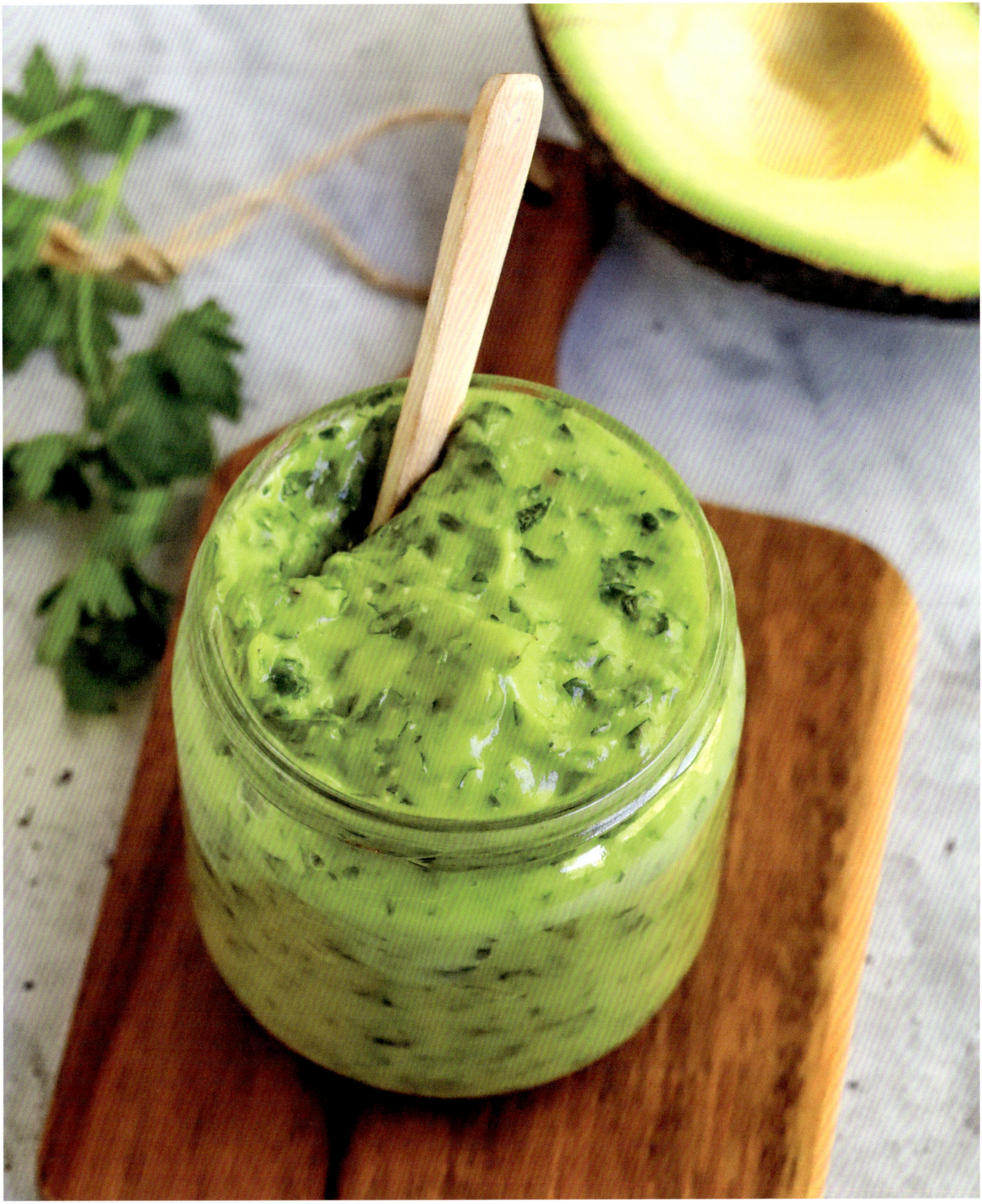

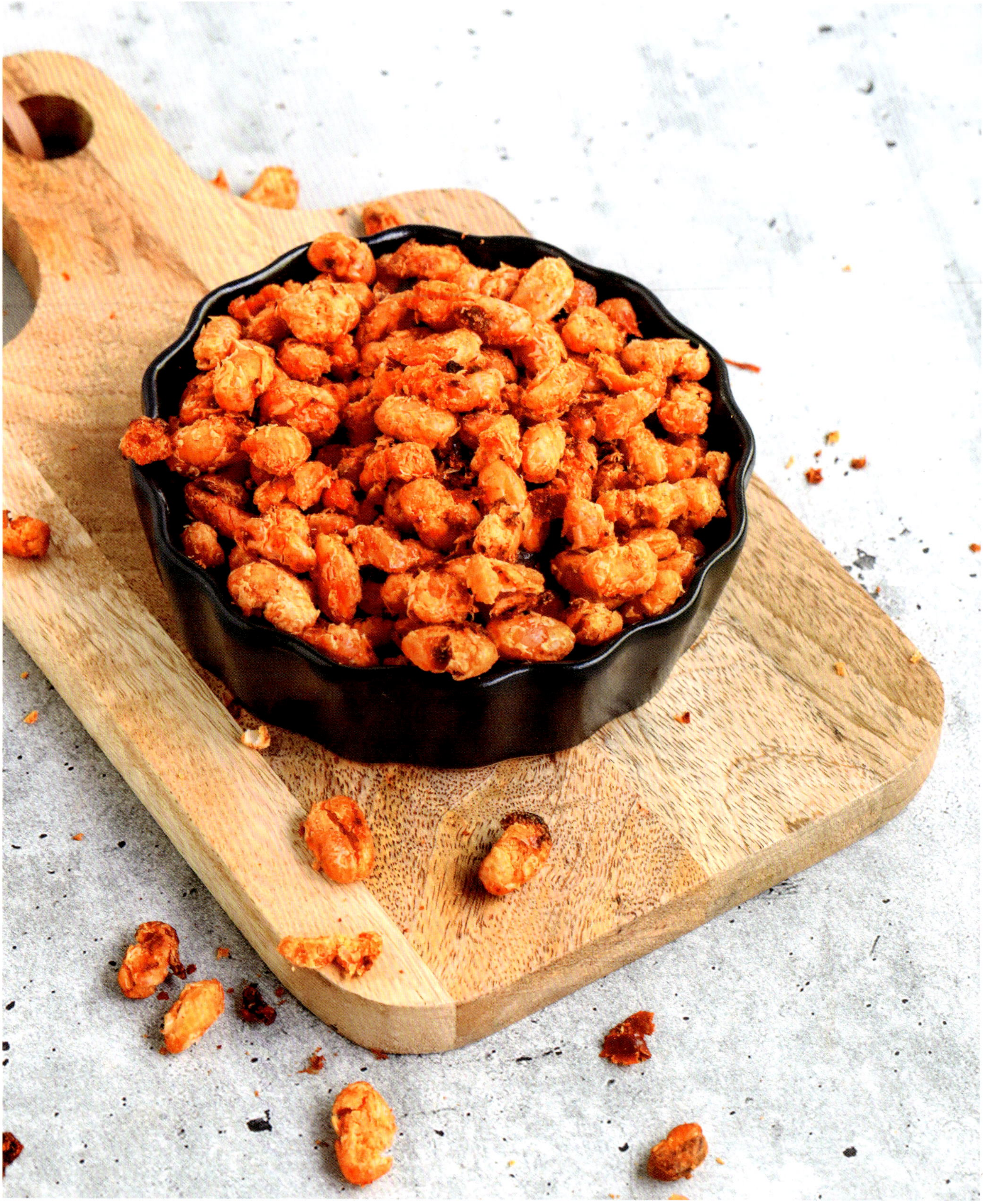

SERVES **4** | **20** MINUTES

HARISSA BUTTER BEANS

INGREDIENTS

14 oz (400 g) can **butter beans**, drained and rinsed
1 tbsp **olive oil**
1 tsp **sea salt**
1 tsp **freshly ground black pepper**
1 tsp **garlic powder**
1 tbsp **harissa paste**
½ tbsp smoked **paprika**

METHOD

- Place all the ingredients into a bowl and stir well to ensure the beans are evenly coated in the mixture.
- Preheat the air fryer to 400°F (200°C). Spread the seasoned butter beans in a single layer in the air fryer basket. Avoid overcrowding to ensure an even cook.
- Air fry for 12–15 minutes, tossing the beans halfway through the cook, until they are golden and crispy.
- Once cooked, add any additional seasoning or flavours if desired. Allow the beans to cool completely before transferring them to an airtight container.
- Storage: Store the air-fried butter beans in the container for 3–5 days at room temperature.

ENERGY: **108** kcal | CARBS: **13** g | PROTEIN: **5** g | FAT: **4** g | FIBRE: **4** g

MINI BLUEBERRY AND LEMON CHEESECAKE

INGREDIENTS

For the base

3.5 oz (100 g) **almonds**
2 oz (55 g) **medjool dates**, pitted
2 tbsp **coconut oil**

For the cheesecake filling

3.5 oz (100 g) **cashews**, soaked overnight, or boiled for 5 minutes
juice of 1 **lemon**
4 tbsp **coconut oil**, melted
3 tbsp **maple syrup**
5.3 oz (150 g) **blueberries**, fresh or frozen

METHOD

- To prepare the base, place the almonds and dates in a food processor. Process until the mixture reaches a fine crumb consistency. Add the coconut oil and continue to blend until well combined.
- Firmly press the mixture into silicone muffin moulds using a glass or your fingers. Place in the freezer while preparing the cheesecake layer.
- Place the drained cashews, lemon juice, melted coconut oil and maple syrup into a food processor and blend until smooth.
- Remove the bases from the freezer. Place a few blueberries on each base and then spoon over the cheesecake mixture.
- Garnish with additional blueberries and place the moulds back in the freezer and freeze for 2–3 hours to set. Remove the cheesecakes from the freezer 1 hour before serving.

ENERGY: **389** kcal | CARBS: **43** g | PROTEIN: **7** g | FIBRE: **5** g | FAT: **21** g

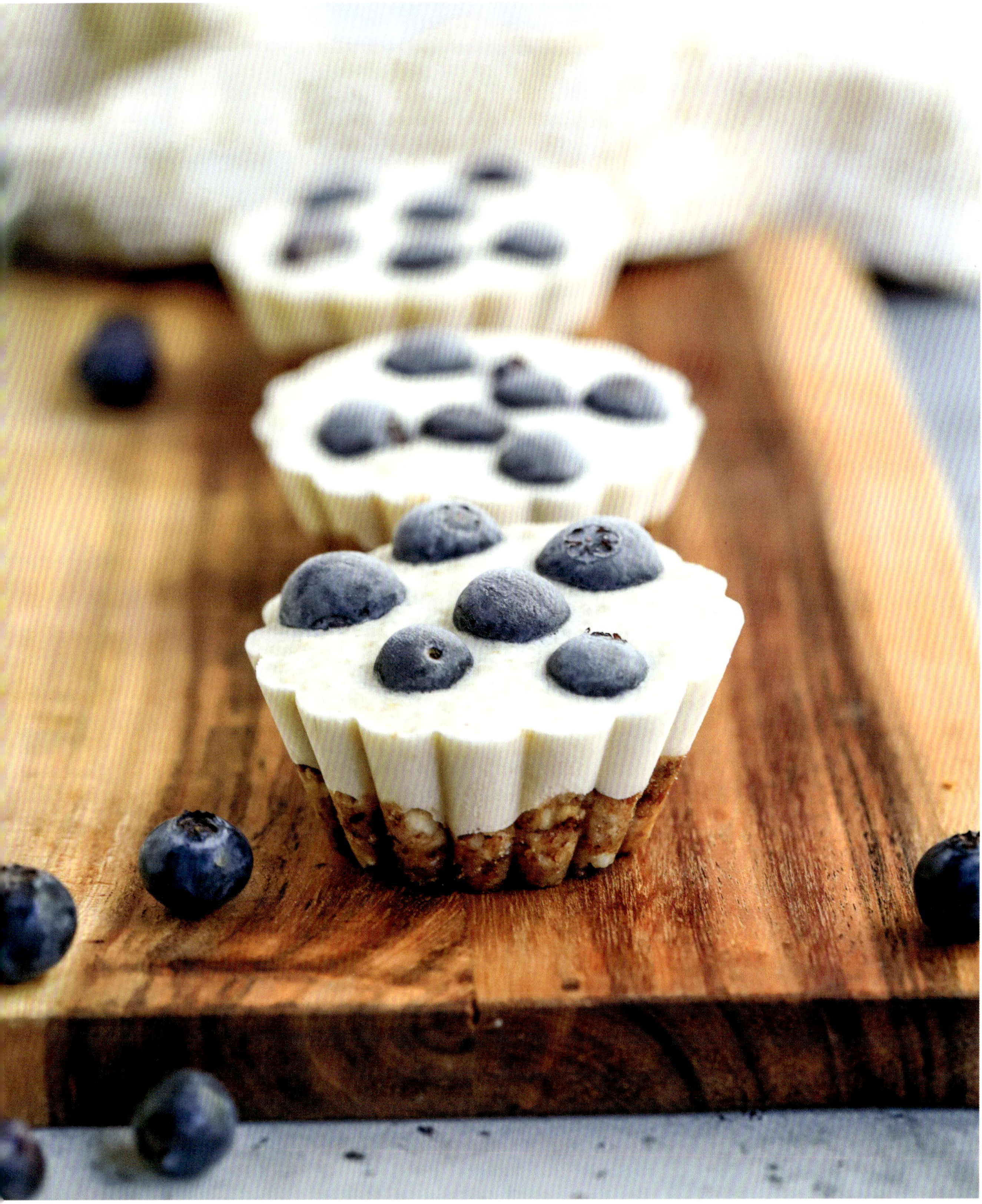

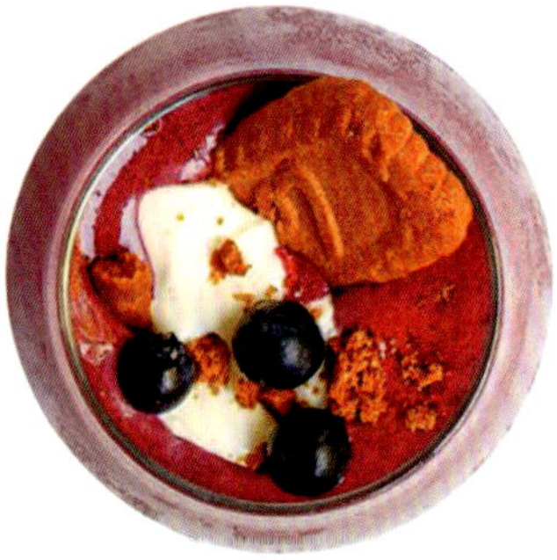

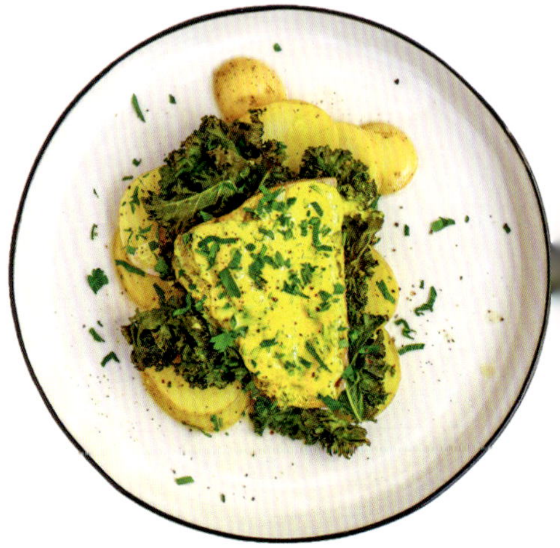

RECIPES WEEK 5

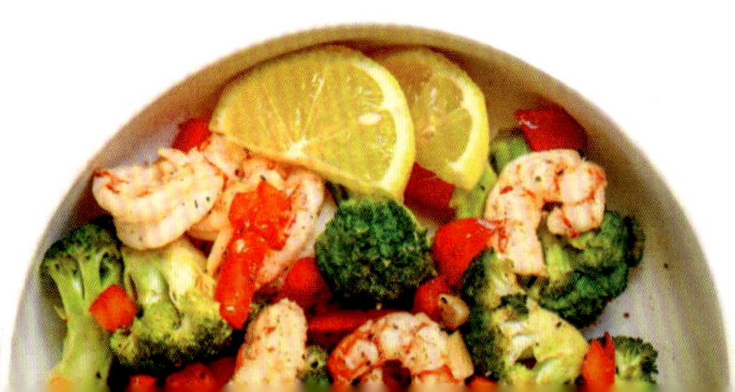

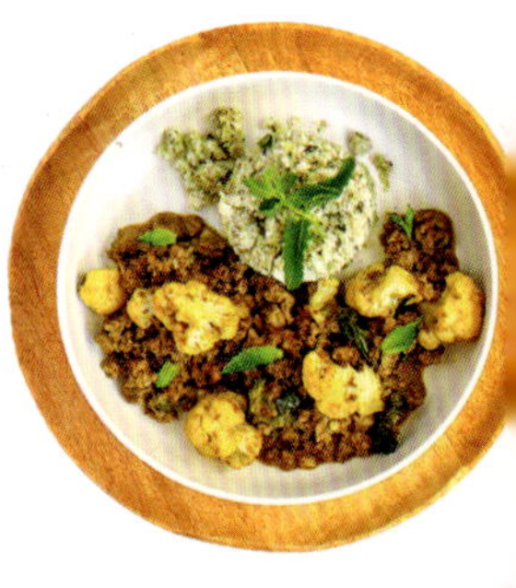

WEEKLY SHOPPING LIST

PRODUCE

1 avocado
2 bananas
4 lemons
2 limes pineapple
1 onion
2 red onions
1 bunch green onions (spring onions)
2 bulbs garlic
2 carrots
3 tomatoes cherry tomatoes
1 red chili
1 red bell pepper
mushrooms
baby spinach
arugula (rocket)
kale
1 head broccoli
1 head of cauliflower
potatoes
basil chives
cilantro (coriander)
dill
mint
parsley
thyme
dried apricots
dried dates
frozen blueberries

PROTEIN

1.8 lb (800 g) 95% lean ground beef (beef mince)
4 oz (115 g) shredded rotisserie chicken (or use leftover roast chicken)
10 oz (280 g) cooked chicken breast
2 lb (900 g) boneless, skinless chicken breasts
1 lb (450 g) raw shrimp
4.2 oz (120 g) hot smoked salmon
1.2 lb (565 g) tuna steak (cut into 4 steaks)
11 eggs milk
unsweetened vanilla flavoured almond milk
Greek yogurt
butter grated/shredded
mozzarella cheese
cheddar cheese
cottage cheese
cream cheese
11.3 oz (320 g) pack shortcrust pastry

STAPLES AND MISC

coconut oil honey
1 x 4.2 oz (120 g) can tuna in water or brine
2 x 14 oz (400 g) can black beans
1 x 14 oz (400 g) can cannellini beans
1 x 7 oz (200 g) can butter beans
1 x 2.6 oz (75 g) can artichoke hearts
1 x 14 oz (400 g) can light coconut milk
jar roasted red peppers
mayonnaise
Dijon mustard
basil
pesto
balsamic vinegar
pasta shells
peanut butter
almond butter
flaky sea salt
vanilla protein powder pack
8 small flour or corn tortillas
2 large flour tortillas
granola (or use granola recipe from this pack)

DRY GOODS

rolled oats
white rice
almonds
peanuts
desiccated coconut
pumpkin seeds
sunflower seeds
dark chocolate chips
vanilla extract
ground coriander
ground cumin
ground turmeric
ground cinnamon
red pepper flakes
jerk seasoning
Italian seasoning
rendang powder (or use rendang paste)
dried thyme

Sample Weekly Meal Planner

	BREAKFAST	LUNCH
Monday	PESTO CHICKEN WRAPS	LEMON AND HERB SALMON PASTA
Tueday	CHICKEN AND SPINACH QUICHE	LEMON AND HERB SALMON PASTA
Wednesday	CHICKEN AND SPINACH QUICHE	SPICED KOFTE WITH CARROT AND YOGURT SALAD
Thursday	BLUEBERRY CHEESECAKE PROTEIN SMOOTHIE	SPICED KOFTE WITH CARROT AND YOGURT SALAD
Friday	FRUIT AND NUT CLUSTER GRANOLA	GARLICKY SHRIMP AND BROCCOLI STIR-FRY
Saturday	FRUIT AND NUT CLUSTER GRANOLA	WHITE BEAN TUNA SALAD
Sunday	PESTO CHICKEN WRAPS	WHITE BEAN TUNA SALAD

SNACK	DINNER
SALTED CINNAMON PROTEIN BARS	RENDANG-SPICED BEEF AND CAULIFLOWER RICE
FRUIT AND NUT CLUSTER GRANOLA	RENDANG-SPICED BEEF AND CAULIFLOWER RICE
PEANUT BUTTER BANANA COTTAGE CHEESE BARK	MEAL PREP JERK CHICKEN AND PINEAPPLE SALSA
PEANUT BUTTER BANANA COTTAGE CHEESE BARK	MEAL PREP JERK CHICKEN AND PINEAPPLE SALSA
BLUEBERRY CHEESECAKE PROTEIN SMOOTHIE	FOIL BAKED CHICKEN AND BUTTER BEANS
SALTED CINNAMON PROTEIN BARS	MEAL OUT – ENJOY!
SALTED CINNAMON PROTEIN BARS	DIJON AND TURMERIC TUNA PARCELS

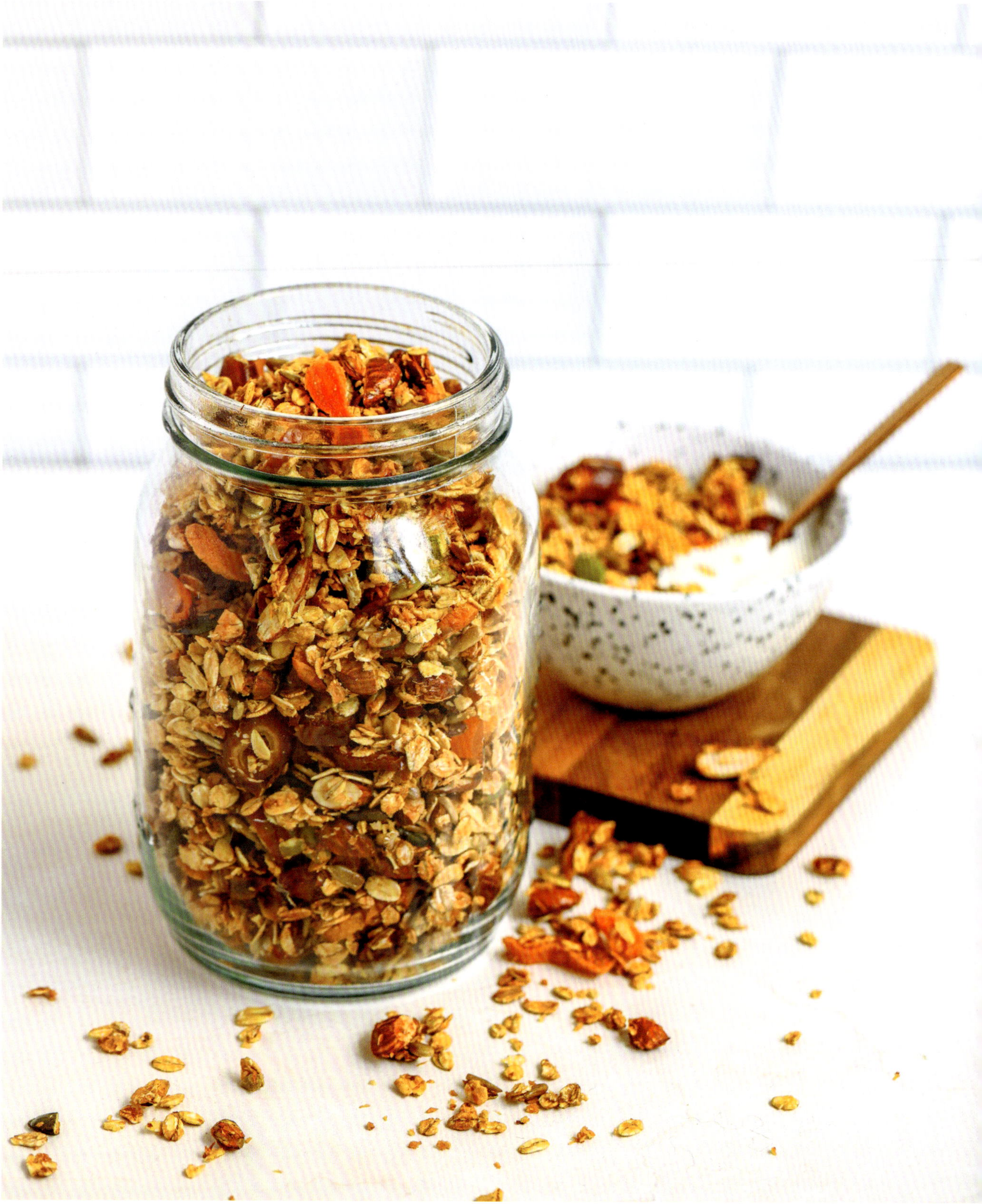

SERVES **16** | **40** MINUTES

FRUIT AND NUT CLUSTER GRANOLA

INGREDIENTS

8 tbsp **honey**
2.6 oz (75 g) **almonds**
10.6 oz (300 g) **rolled oats**
1.4 oz (40 g) **sunflower seeds**
1.4 oz (40 g) **pumpkin seeds**
1 oz (30 g) **desiccated coconut**, unsweetened
1.8 oz (50 g) **dates (pitted)**
3.5 oz (100 g) **dried apricots**

METHOD

- Preheat the oven to 300°F (150°C). Warm the honey in a small saucepan over low heat until it becomes runny.
- Roughly chop the almonds, then spread them over a large baking sheet along with the rolled oats, sunflower seeds, pumpkin seeds and desiccated coconut.
- Drizzle the warm honey evenly over the oat mixture and stir until well combined. Place in the oven and bake for 20 minutes, stirring occasionally.
- Meanwhile, pit and chop the dates and the dried apricots into small bite-sized pieces.
- After 20 minutes add the chopped dried fruits to the baking sheet and stir to combine. Return to the oven for 10 minutes. Avoid stirring too much during this time so that the granola forms clusters.
- Remove the granola from the oven and set aside to cool completely before breaking into chunks.
- Storage: Store in an airtight jar or container, on the countertop, for up to 1 month.
- **Serving suggestion:** Serve with yogurt and fresh or poached seasonal fruit (not included in nutritional breakdown).

ENERGY: **203** kcal | CARBS: **30** g | PROTEIN: **5** g | FAT: **7** g

SERVES **4** | **25** MINUTES

HEARTY MEXICAN **BREAKFAST TACOS**

INGREDIENTS

3 ripe **tomatoes**, finely diced
2 **roasted red peppers** (from a jar), drained, finely diced
4 **green onions**, finely sliced
½–1 **lime**, juiced
14 oz (400 g) **canned black beans**
8 small **flour** or **corn tortillas**
1 tbsp **butter**
8 large **free-range eggs**
coriander, chopped, to garnish

METHOD

- Place the tomatoes, roasted red peppers and green onions in a large bowl, squeeze over the juice from ½ a lime and drizzle over 1 tablespoon of extra virgin olive oil. Season with salt and pepper, then taste, adding more seasoning or lime juice if needed. Set aside.
- Place 2 teaspoons of olive oil in a small pot over low-medium heat. Add the black beans, season with salt, and gently heat through, stirring occasionally.
- Heat a dry skillet over medium heat. Toast each tortilla individually on both sides until slightly charred and warmed through. Once toasted, cover the tortillas with a clean tea towel or wrap them in foil, to keep warm.
- In a separate frying pan, heat 4 teaspoons of olive oil with the butter over medium heat. Fry the eggs until the whites are set but the yolks remain soft and runny (cook longer for firmer yolks).
- Place two tortillas on each plate. Top with a spoonful of warmed black beans, a generous portion of salsa, and top with fried eggs. Garnish with chopped coriander if desire.

ENERGY: **441** kcal | CARBS: **41** g | PROTEIN: **22** g | FAT: **21** g

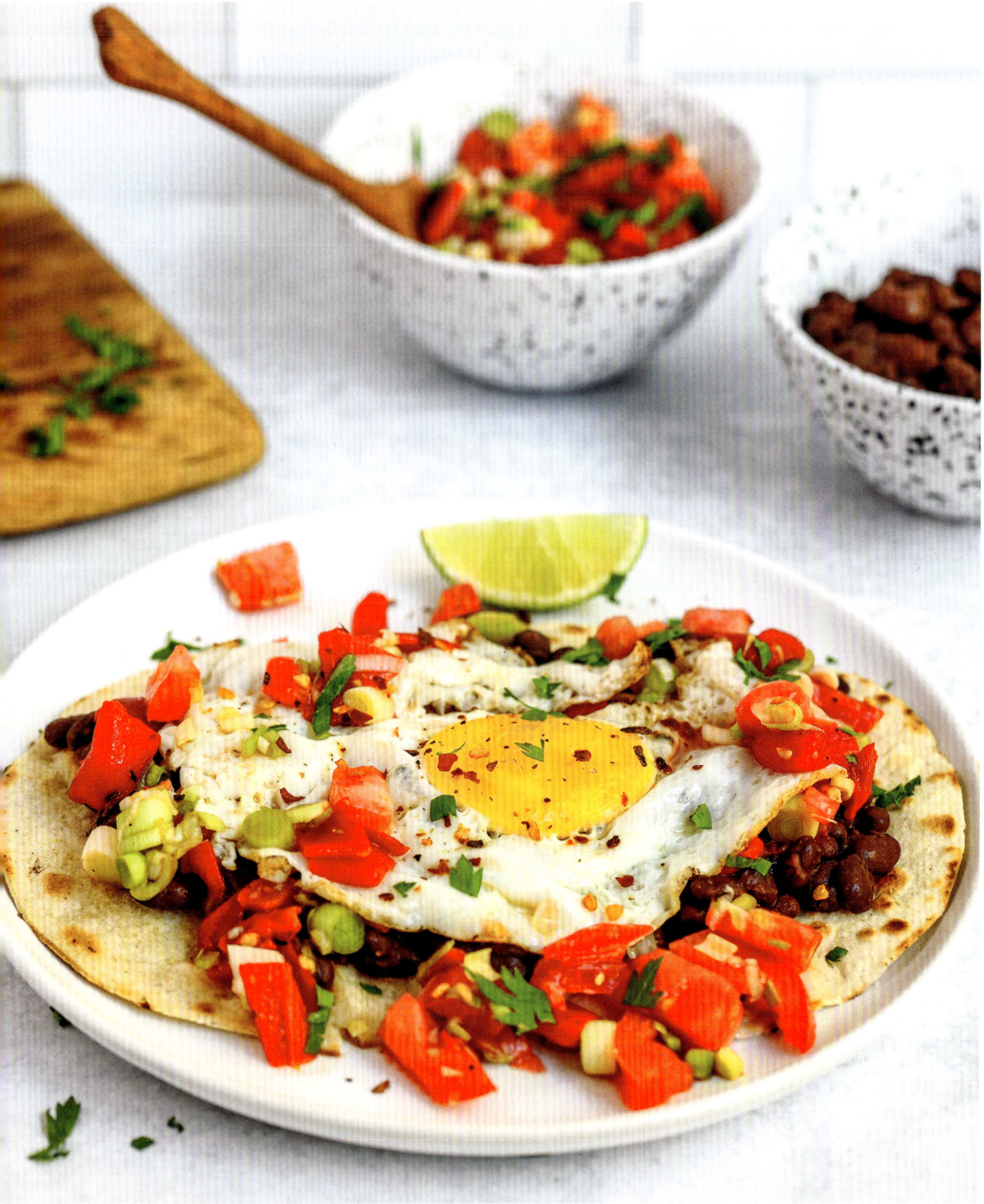

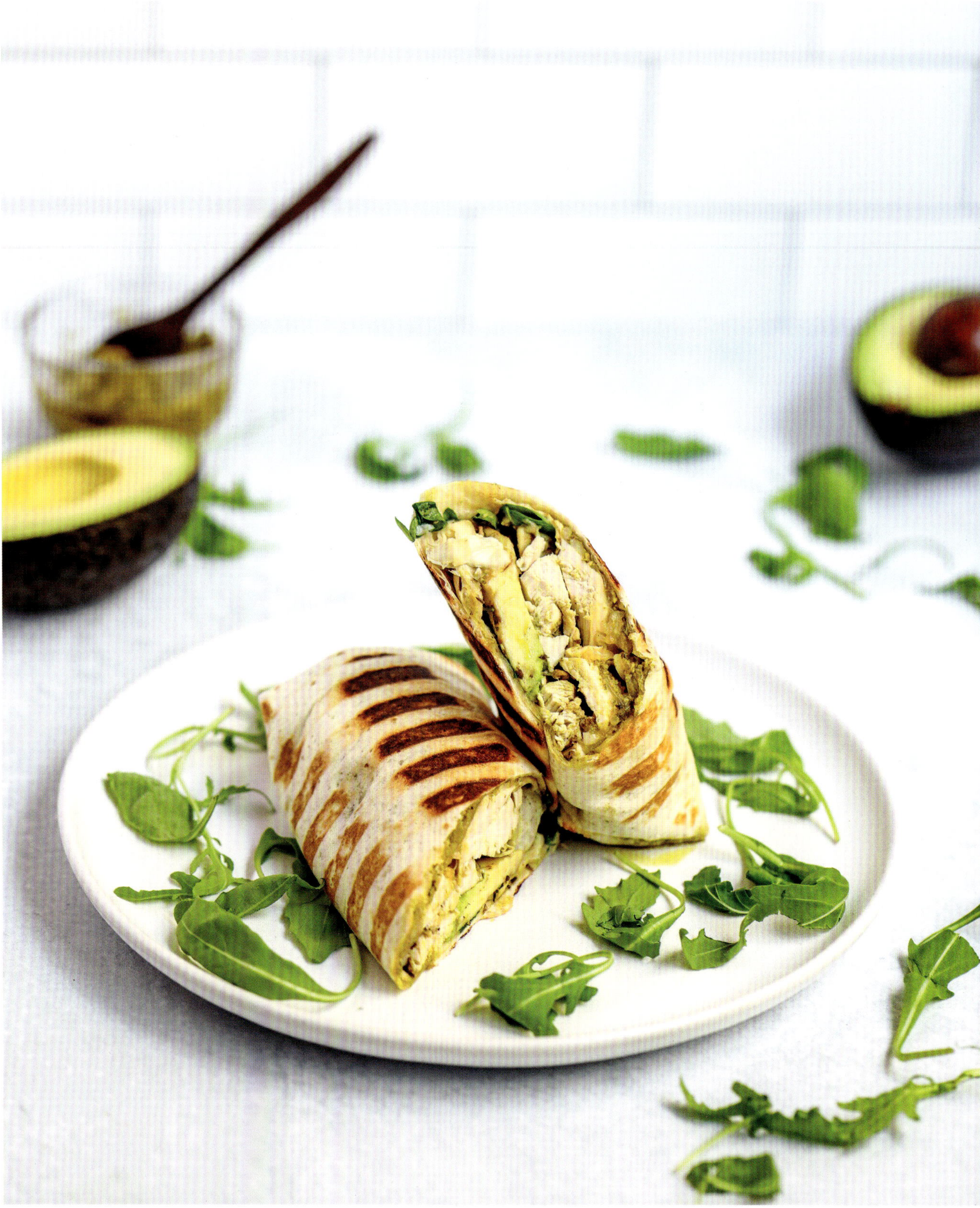

SERVES **2** | **15** MINUTES

PESTO CHICKEN WRAPS

INGREDIENTS

2 large **flour tortillas**
1 oz (30 g) **grated mozzarella**
2 tbsp **basil pesto**
4 oz (115 g) **cooked chicken breast**
2.6 oz (75 g) **canned artichoke hearts**, chopped
1 **avocado**, pitted and sliced
2 tsp **Italian seasoning**
1 oz (30 g) **arugula (rocket)**

METHOD

- In the centre of each tortilla, layer mozzarella, basil pesto, shredded chicken, artichoke hearts and sliced avocado.
- Sprinkle with Italian seasoning and top with a handful of arugula.
- Preheat a dry grill pan or skillet over medium high heat. Fold the sides of the tortilla inward and roll up like a burrito.
- Grill the wraps for 4–6 minutes on each side or until golden brown and crispy. Serve warm.

ENERGY: **347** kcal	CARBS: **19** g	PROTEIN: **25** g	FAT: **19** g

SERVES **6** | **1** HOUR **40** MINUTES

CHICKEN AND SPINACH **QUICHE**

INGREDIENTS

11.3 oz (320 g) **shortcrust pastry**
7 large **eggs**, beaten
5 oz (150 ml) **milk**
10 oz (280 g) **cooked chicken breast**, diced
2.6 oz (75 g) **baby spinach**, shopped
2 oz (35 g) **cheddar cheese**, shredded
4 oz (115 g) **mushrooms**, sliced
½ tsp dried **thyme**

METHOD

- Preheat the oven to 400°F (200°C). Prepare a round springform pan or dish and place on a baking sheet.
- Press the dough firmly into the bottom and sides of the dish. Fold or crimp the edges of the dough as desired.
- If necessary, precook the pastry according to instructions on packaging.
- In a large mixing bowl, lightly beat the eggs with the milk. Add the diced chicken, spinach, cheese, mushrooms, 1 tsp salt, ⅛ tsp black pepper, and thyme. Stir to combine.
- Once the crust is par-baked, remove from the oven and pour the egg mixture into the crust. Cover the exposed edges of the pie crust with foil to prevent over-browning.
- Place the quiche dish (still on the baking sheet) on the middle oven rack and bake for 50–60 minutes, or until the eggs are set and a knife inserted in the centre comes out clean.
- Remove quiche from the oven and set aside to cool for 10–15 minutes before slicing and serving.
- **Serving suggestion:** Pair with a crisp green salad.

ENERGY: **433** kcal | PROTEIN: **28** g | CARBS: **24** g | FAT: **25** g

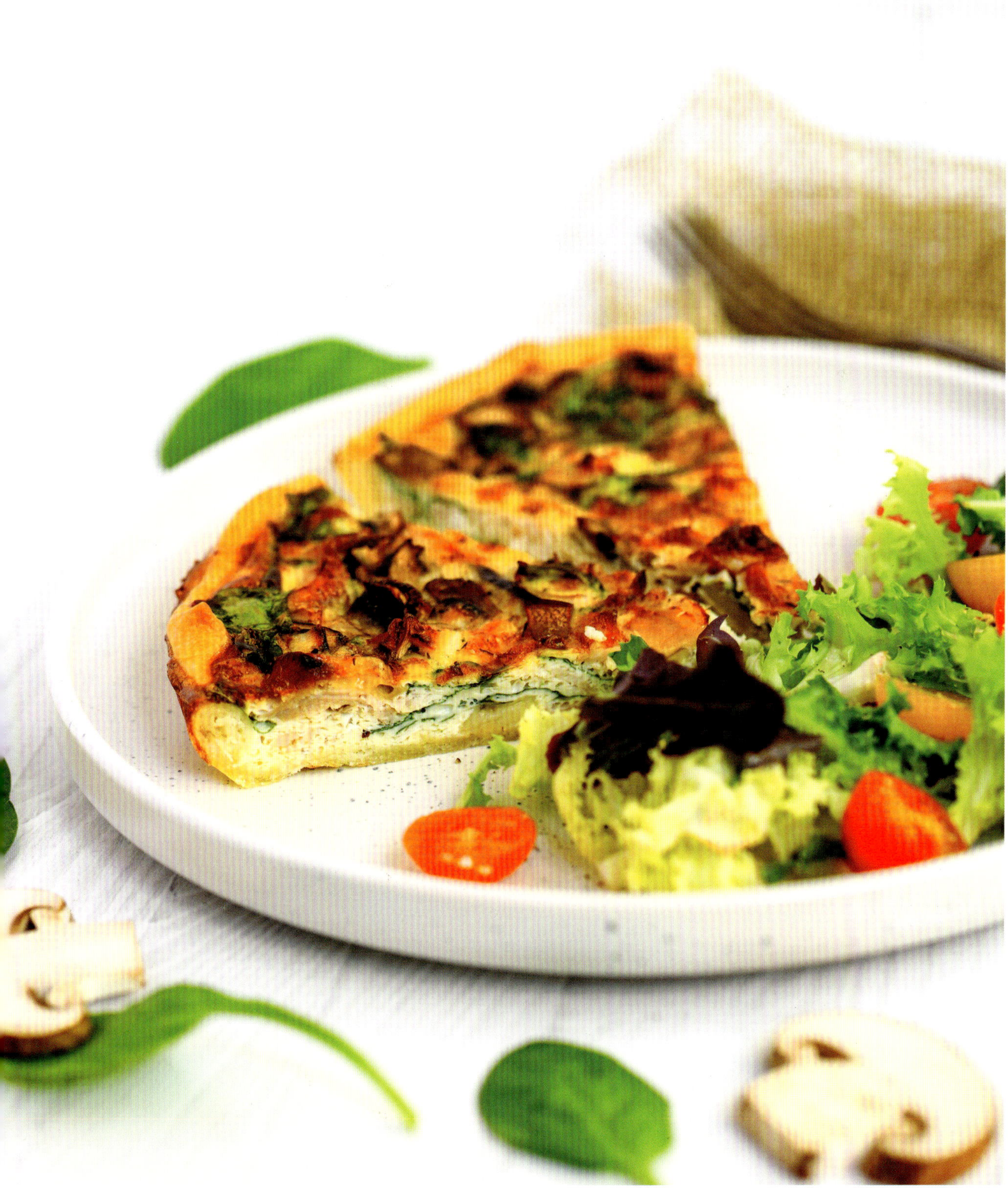

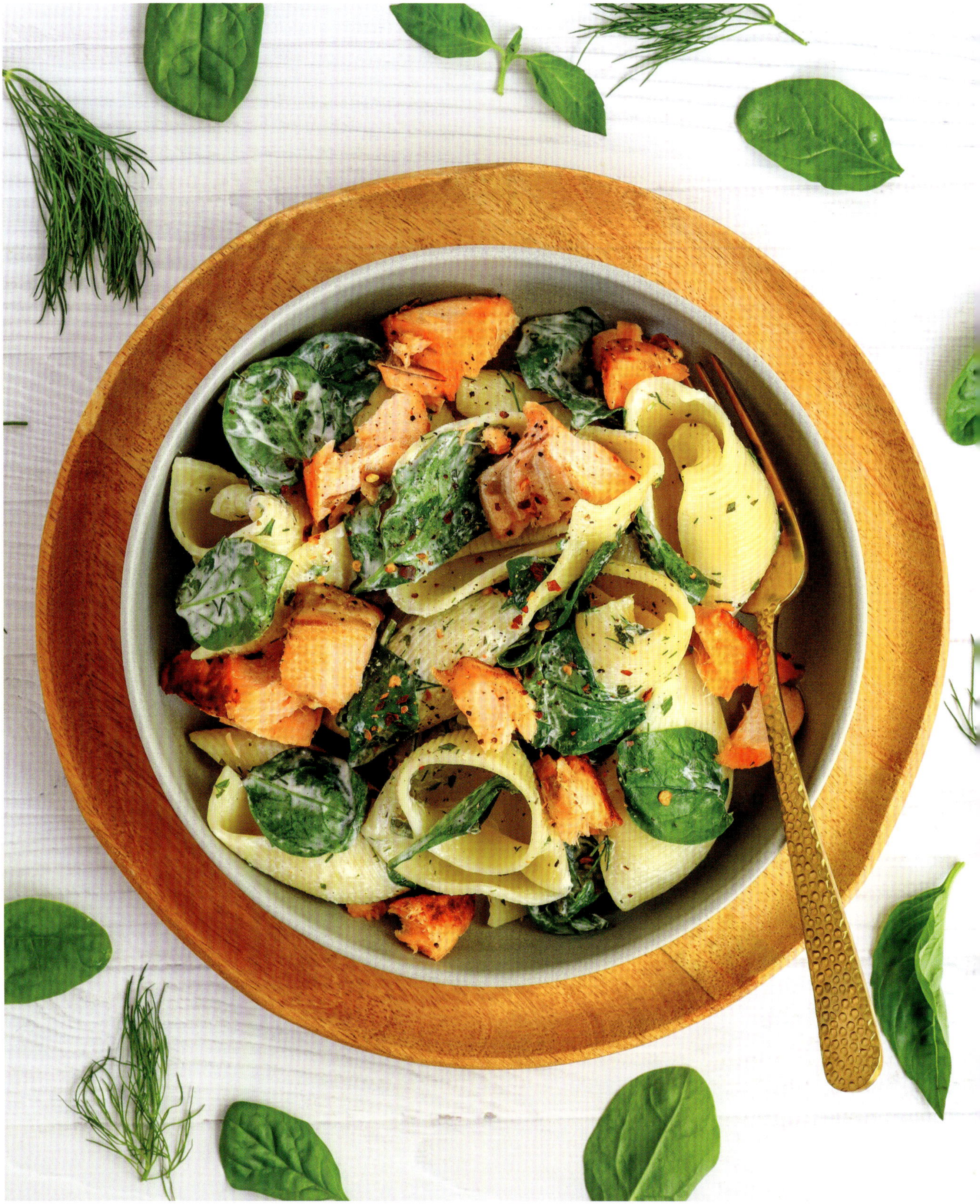

SERVES **2** | **15** MINUTES

LEMON AND HERB SALMON PASTA

INGREDIENTS

7 oz (200 g) **pasta shells**
2 tbsp **fresh parsley**, chopped
2 tbsp **fresh basil**, chopped
2 tbsp **fresh chives**, chopped
2 tbsp **fresh dill**, chopped
3.5 oz (100 g) **Greek yogurt**
juice of 2 **lemons**
2.1 oz (60 g) **baby spinach**
4.2 oz (120 g) **hot-smoked salmon**, broken into large pieces

METHOD

- Cook the pasta according to the package instructions until al dente. Drain and set aside.
- Place the fresh herbs into a small bowl, along with Greek yogurt and lemon juice. Season with salt and black pepper to taste.
- Toss the cooked pasta with the herby yogurt mixture until evenly coated. Gently fold in the baby spinach. Adjust seasoning with additional salt and pepper if needed.
- Serve the pasta lukewarm, topped with the pieces of hot-smoked salmon.

ENERGY: **466** kcal | CARBS: **78** g | PROTEIN: **25** g | FAT: **6** g

SERVES **4** | **20** MINUTES

SPICED KOFTE WITH CARROT AND YOGURT SALAD

INGREDIENTS

1 yellow **onion**, diced
2 **garlic** cloves, minced
2½ tbsp **fresh parsley**, chopped
14 oz (400 g) **95% lean ground beef**
2 tbsp **quick oats**
1 tsp **ground coriander**
1 tsp **ground cumin**
2 **carrots**, peeled and grated
2 **green onions**, sliced
2.1 oz (60 g) **Greek yogurt**
2 tbsp **balsamic vinegar**
parsley, chopped, to garnish

METHOD

- Place the onion, garlic, parsley, ground beef, oats, coriander and cumin in a large bowl and season with salt and pepper. Mix well to combine and, using your hands, shape the mixture into small, elongated patties (kofte).
- Heat 1 tablespoon of olive oil in a skillet over medium-high heat. Sauté the kofte for 5 minutes, turning occasionally, until golden brown and crispy on all sides.
- Mix the carrots, green onions, yogurt, balsamic vinegar, and 2 tbsp olive oil in a bowl. Season with salt and pepper to taste, and set aside.
- Once the kofte is cooked, serve alongside the carrot salad, garnished with chopped parsley.

ENERGY: **325** kcal	CARBS: **11** g	PROTEIN: **23** g	FAT: **21** g

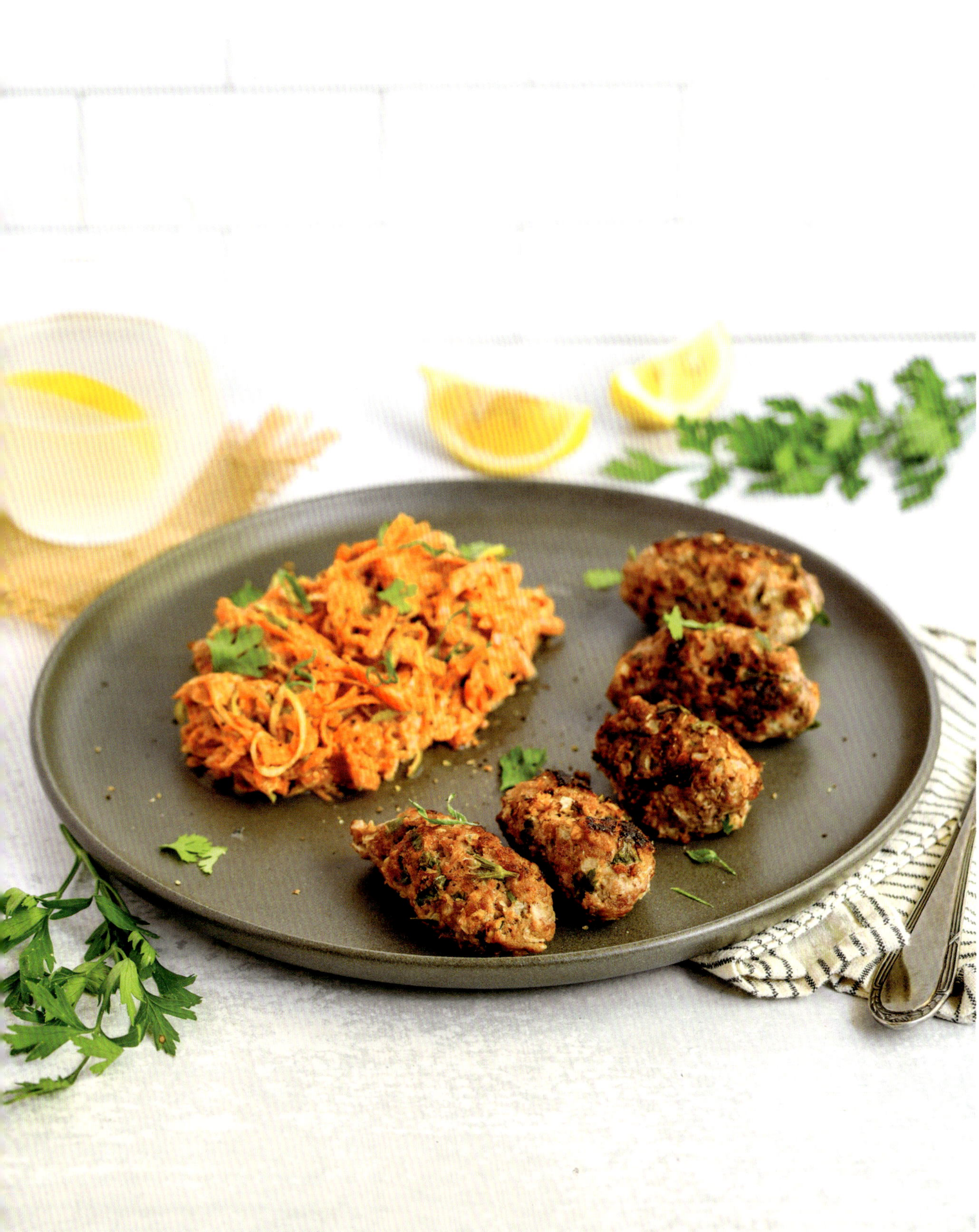

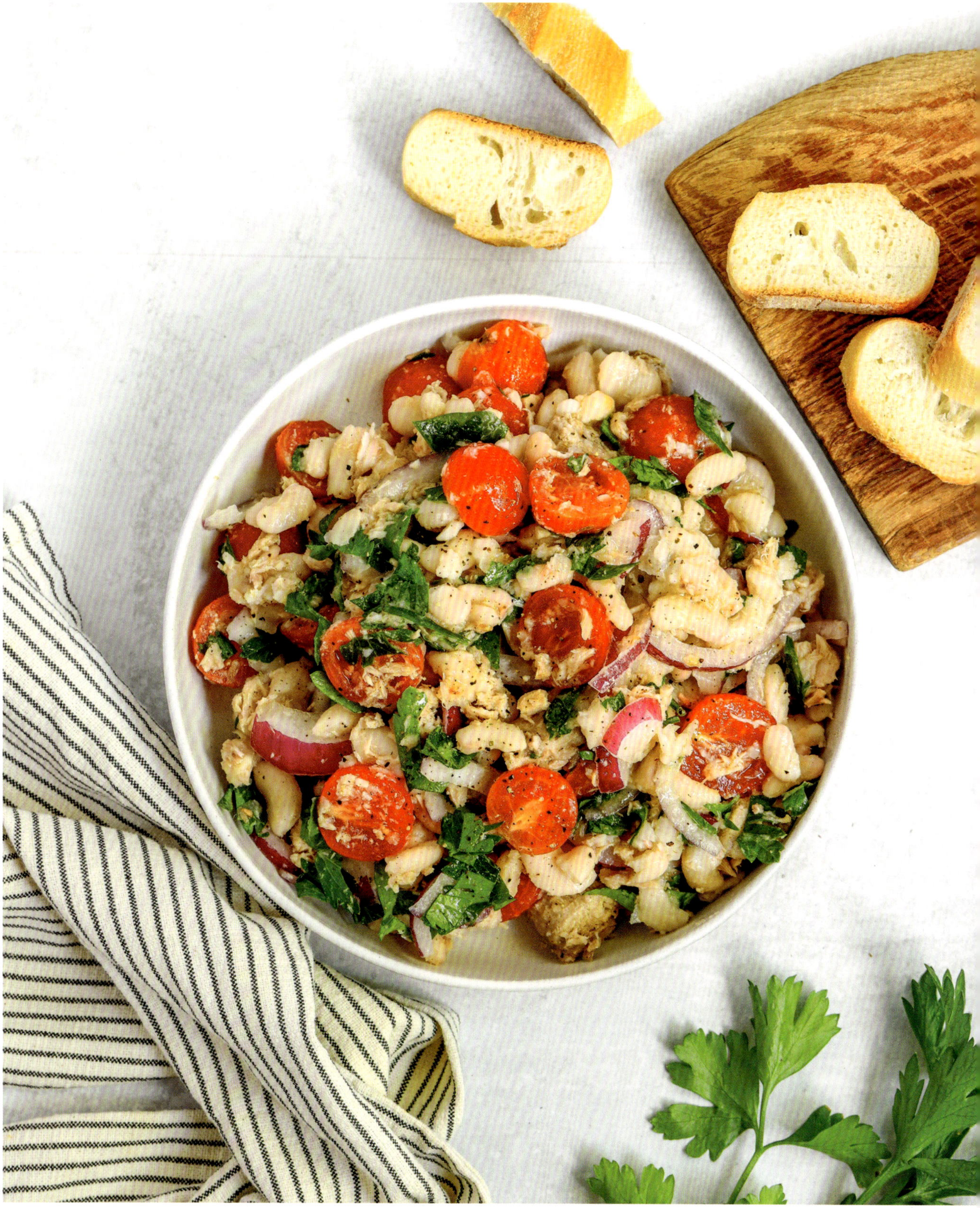

SERVES **2** | **15** MINUTES

WHITE BEAN TUNA **SALAD**

INGREDIENTS

½ **red onion**, thinly sliced
2½ tbsp **fresh parsley**, chopped
10.6 oz (300 g) **canned cannellini beans**, drained
4.2 oz (120 g) **canned tuna** (in water or brine), drained
7 oz (200 g) **cherry tomatoes**, halved

METHOD

- Place the onion, parsley, cannellini beans, tuna and tomatoes in a large bowl. Drizzle with 2 tbsp olive oil and 2 tbsp white wine vinegar.
- Season to taste with salt and pepper and toss everything together until well combined. Refrigerate until ready to serve.

ENERGY: **351** kcal | CARBS: **32** g | PROTEIN: **22** g | FAT: **15** g

SERVES **4** | **20** MINUTES

GARLICKY SHRIMP AND BROCCOLI STIR-FRY

INGREDIENTS

6 cloves **garlic**, sliced, divided

1 head **broccoli**, cut into small florets

½ **red bell pepper**, diced

1 lb (450 g) **raw shrimp**, peeled and deveined

1 tsp **lemon juice**, plus extra to taste

METHOD

- Heat 1 tbsp of olive oil in a large pot over medium heat. Add half of the sliced garlic and cook for 1 minute.
- Add the broccoli, red bell pepper, and ¼ teaspoon each of salt and pepper. Cover and cook, stirring occasionally. If the pot becomes dry, add 1 tablespoon of water. Cook for 3–5 minutes, until the vegetables are tender. Transfer the vegetables to a bowl and keep warm.
- Increase the heat to medium-high and add 1 tbsp of olive oil to the pot. Add the remaining garlic and cook for 1 minute.
- Add the shrimp and ¼ teaspoon each of salt and pepper. Cook for 3–5 minutes, stirring frequently, until the shrimp are just cooked through.
- Return the broccoli mixture to the pot, stir in the lemon juice. Taste and adjust seasoning with additional salt, pepper, or lemon juice if needed. Serve immediately.

ENERGY: **232** kcal	CARBS: **13** g	PROTEIN: **27** g	FAT: **8** g

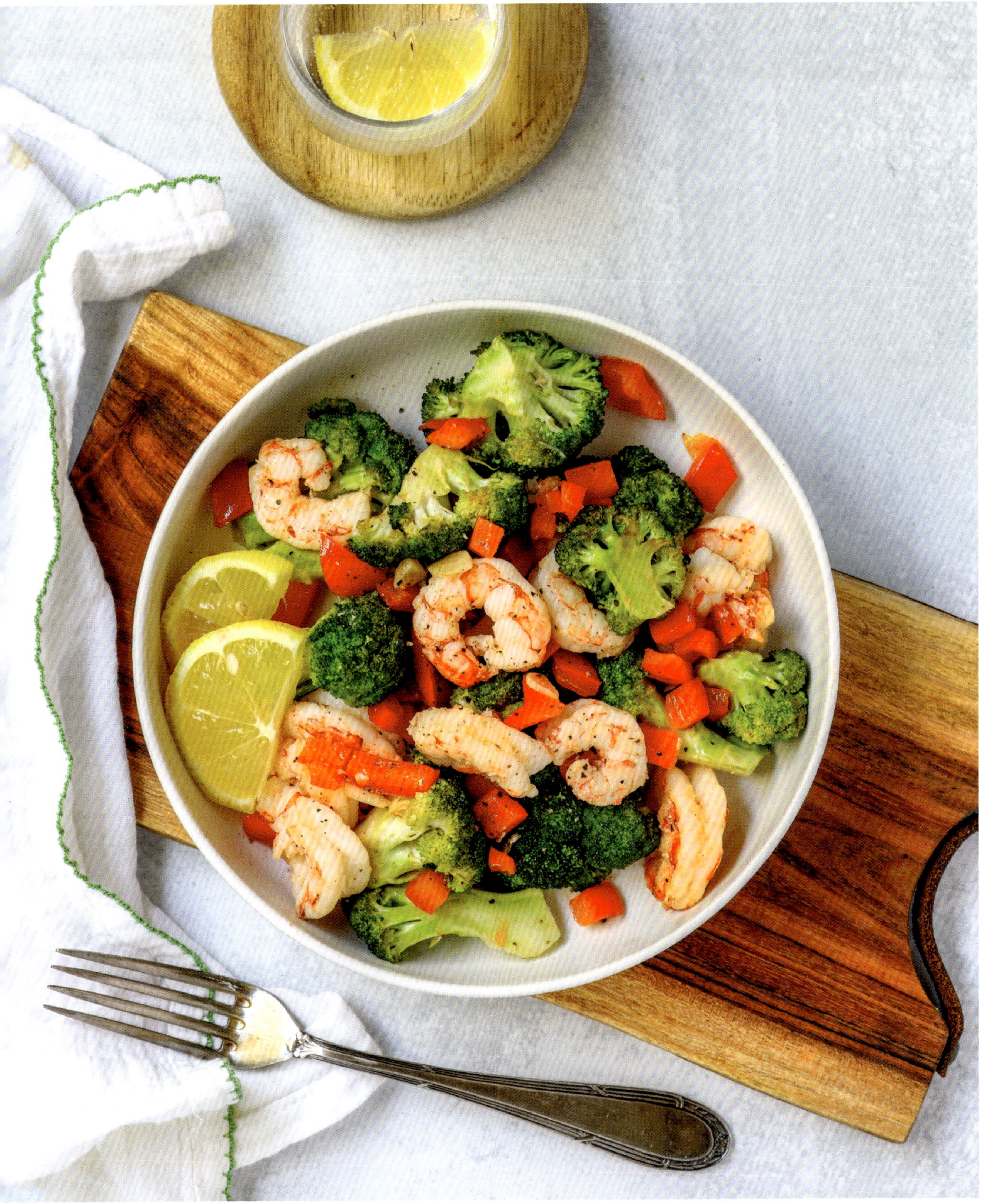

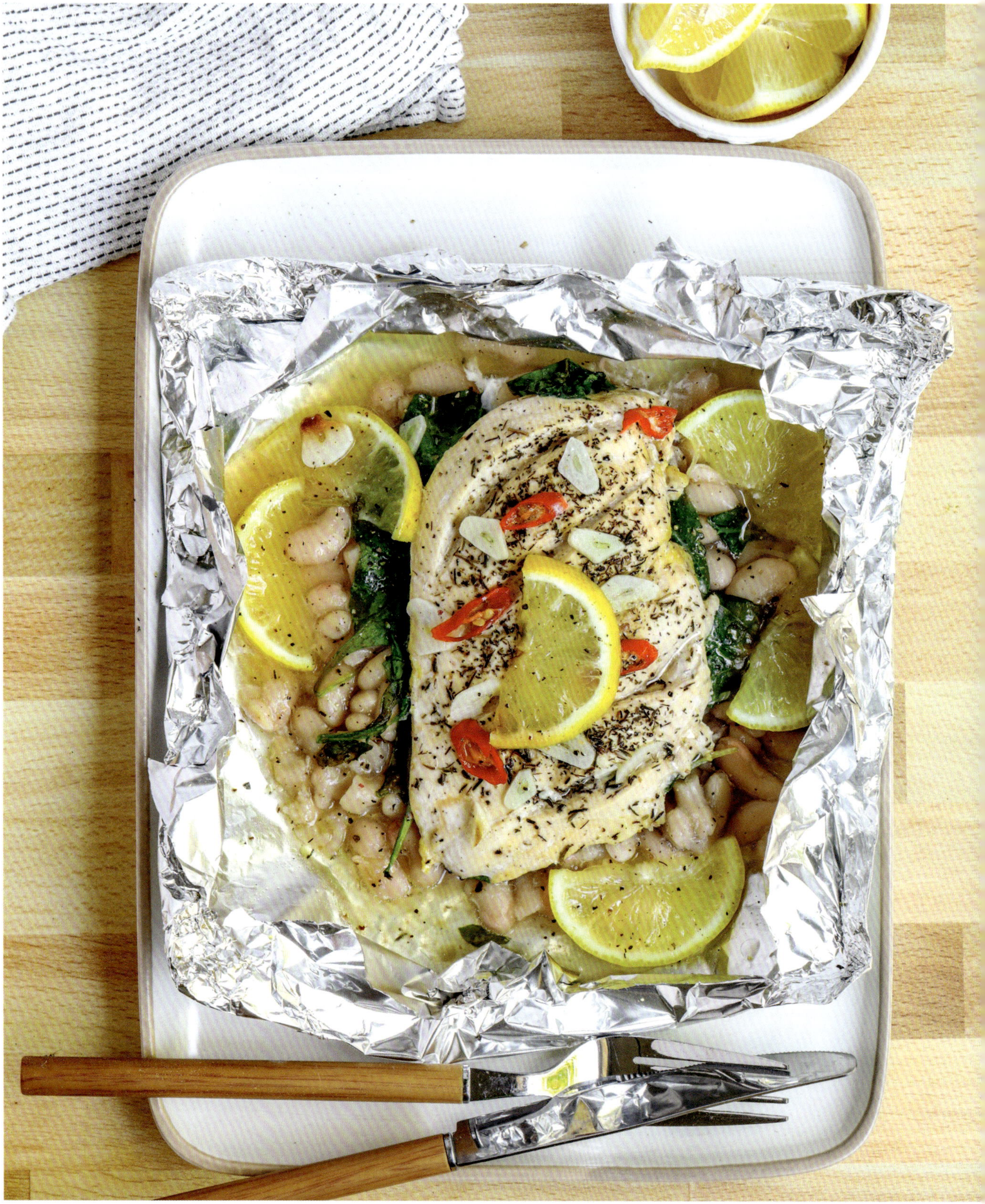

SERVES **2** | **25** MINUTES

FOIL BAKED CHICKEN AND BUTTER BEANS

INGREDIENTS

7 oz (200 g) **canned butter beans**, drain retaining some juice
2.1 oz (60 g) **baby spinach**
2 x **boneless, skinless chicken breast** (5.3 oz (150 g) each)
2 sprigs of **fresh thyme**
2 cloves **garlic**, finely sliced
1 **red chili**, finely sliced (deseed if preferred)
1 **lemon**, finely sliced

METHOD

- Preheat the oven to 430°F (220°C). Lay out two large sheets of thick tin foil, about 24" (60 cm) in length.
- On one half of each sheet of foil, pile half of the butter beans, along with some of the juice from the jar or can. Scatter half the spinach over the beans and season with sea salt and black pepper. Drizzle with ½ tablespoon of olive oil and 1 tbsp red wine vinegar.
- Score the chicken breast widthways at ½" (1 cm) intervals, cutting about halfway through the meat. Season the chicken with salt and pepper, then place the chicken breast over the spinach. Pick the thyme leaves off the sprigs and sprinkle over the chicken.
- Divide the garlic, chili and lemon over each chicken breast. Drizzle everything with 1½ tbsp olive oil.
- Fold the foil over the ingredients, and tightly roll the edges to seal the packets completely.
- Carefully transfer the foil packets to a baking sheet and place on the middle shelf of the oven, and bake for 15 minutes, or until the chicken is cooked through.
- Once done, remove from the oven and set the packets aside to steam for 5 minutes before opening.

ENERGY: **442** kcal | CARBS: **27** g | PROTEIN: **43** g | FAT: **18** g

SERVES **4** | **55** MINUTES

MEAL PREP JERK CHICKEN AND PINEAPPLE **SALSA**

INGREDIENTS

21.1 oz (600 g) **cooked rice**

For the pineapple black bean salsa

10.9 oz (310 g) **pineapple**, diced
8.4 oz (240 g) **canned black beans**, rinsed
½ **red onion**, finely diced
0.5 oz (15 g) **cilantro**, chopped (coriander)
1 **lime**
1 pinch of **crushed red pepper** (optional)

For the jerk chicken

1 tbsp **jerk seasoning**
1.1 lb (600 g) **boneless, skinless chicken breasts**

METHOD

- Place the pineapple, black beans, red onion and cilantro in a large bowl. Squeeze the juice of half a lime over the ingredients. Season with salt and red pepper flakes, and stir to combine. Set the remaining half of the lime aside to cut into wedges for serving.
- Rub jerk seasoning evenly over both sides of the chicken breasts.
- Heat 1 tbsp of oil in a large skillet over medium heat. Cook the chicken for 7 minutes on each side, or until the chicken is browned and fully cooked. Slice the chicken into ½" (1 cm) wide strips.
- Serve 7 oz (200 g) of rice per plate, or meal prep container. Top each serving with 7 oz (200 g) of salsa, and add a few strips of jerk chicken. Add a wedge of lime to each serving.

ENERGY: **560** kcal | CARBS: **77** g | PROTEIN: **45** g | FAT: **8** g

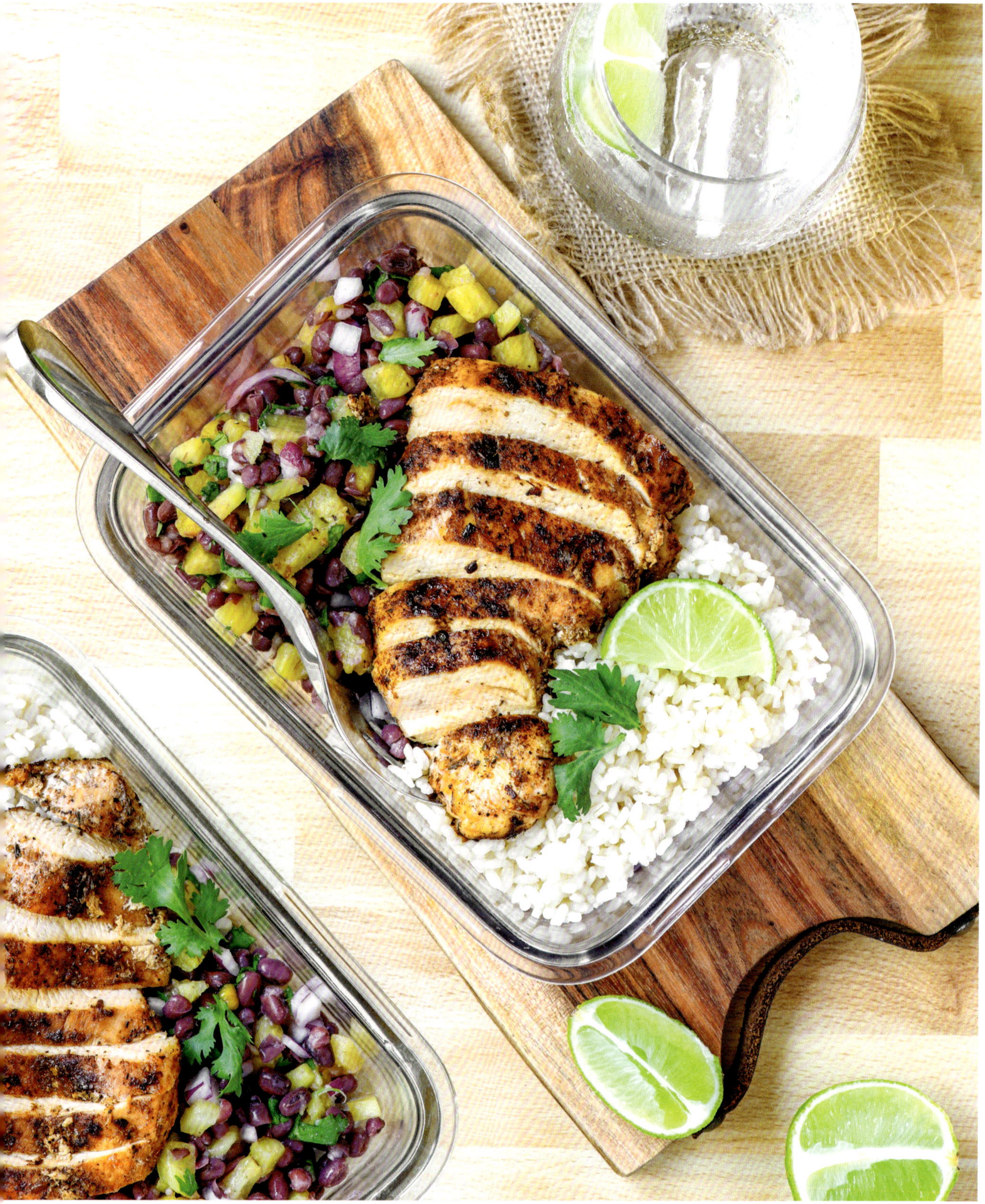

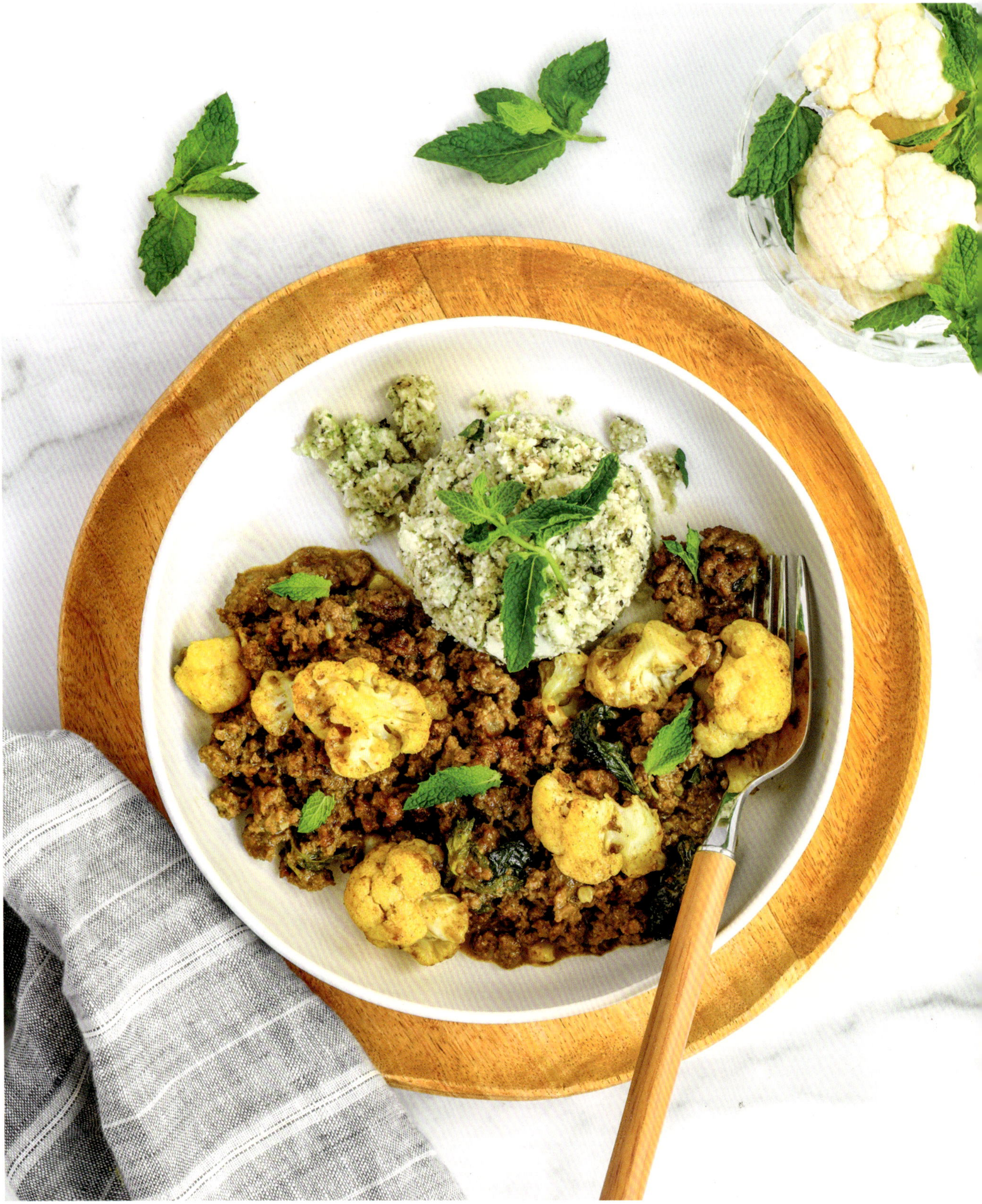

SERVES **4** | **49** MINUTES

RENDANG-SPICED BEEF AND CAULIFLOWER RICE

INGREDIENTS

1.1 lb (500 g) **95% lean ground beef**

1 head of **cauliflower**

1 heaped tsp **rendang powder**

½ oz (15 g) **fresh mint**, plus extra to garnish

14 oz (400 g) can **light coconut milk**

METHOD

- Heat 1 tbsp of olive oil in a large pan over a high heat. Add the beef, stirring regularly and breaking it up, until cooked through.
- Remove and discard the tough outer cauliflower leaves. Place the tender leaves in a food processor.
- Halve the cauliflower, cutting one half into florets and adding to the beef.
- Cut the second half into florets, and place into the food processor along with the stalk.
- Stir the rendang powder into the beef and cauliflower, cooking for 10 minutes until crispy.
- Meanwhile, add half of the mint, and seasoning to the food processor along with the cauliflower, and process to form cauliflower rice. Place the mixture into a bowl and microwave for 4–5 minutes.
- Add the remaining mint to the beef, then pour in coconut milk and half a can of water. Simmer for 5 minutes. Taste and adjust seasoning with salt and pepper.
- Serve the beef with the cauliflower rice on the side, garnished with mint leaves.

ENERGY: **359** kcal | CARBS: **10** g | PROTEIN: **28** g | FAT: **23** g

DIJON AND TURMERIC TUNA PARCELS

INGREDIENTS

4 tbsp **mayonnaise**
1 tbsp **fresh parsley**, chopped
2 tsp **Dijon mustard**
1 tsp **honey**
½ tsp **ground turmeric**
8 oz (225 g) **potatoes**, sliced (about ⅛"/ ¼ cm thick)
5 oz (140 g) **kale**, chopped
1.2 lb (565 g) **tuna steak** (cut into 4 steaks roughly 1" (2½ cm) thick)

METHOD

- Preheat the oven to 450°F (230°C). Cut 4 large sheets of parchment paper (16"x12" / 40x30 cm each).
- Combine mayonnaise, parsley, Dijon mustard, honey and turmeric in a small bowl.
- Fold each parchment sheet in half, then open. Divide the potato slices evenly among the sheets. Season the potatoes with ¼ teaspoon of salt and ⅛ teaspoon of black pepper.
- Add an equal amount of kale to each parcel, then place a piece of tuna on top. Season the tuna with ¼ teaspoon of salt and black pepper. Brush the tuna with the mayonnaise mixture.
- Fold the parchment over and tightly seal the edges with small folds. Arrange the packets on a baking sheet.
- Bake for 10–15 minutes, until the tuna is cooked through. Carefully open one packet to check done (take care with steam). Set the packets aside to rest for 3 minutes.
- To serve, cut an X in the top of each packet and gently fold to open. Transfer to a plate or serve straight from the parcel.

ENERGY: 308 kcal	CARBS: 13 g	PROTEIN: 37 g	FAT: 12 g

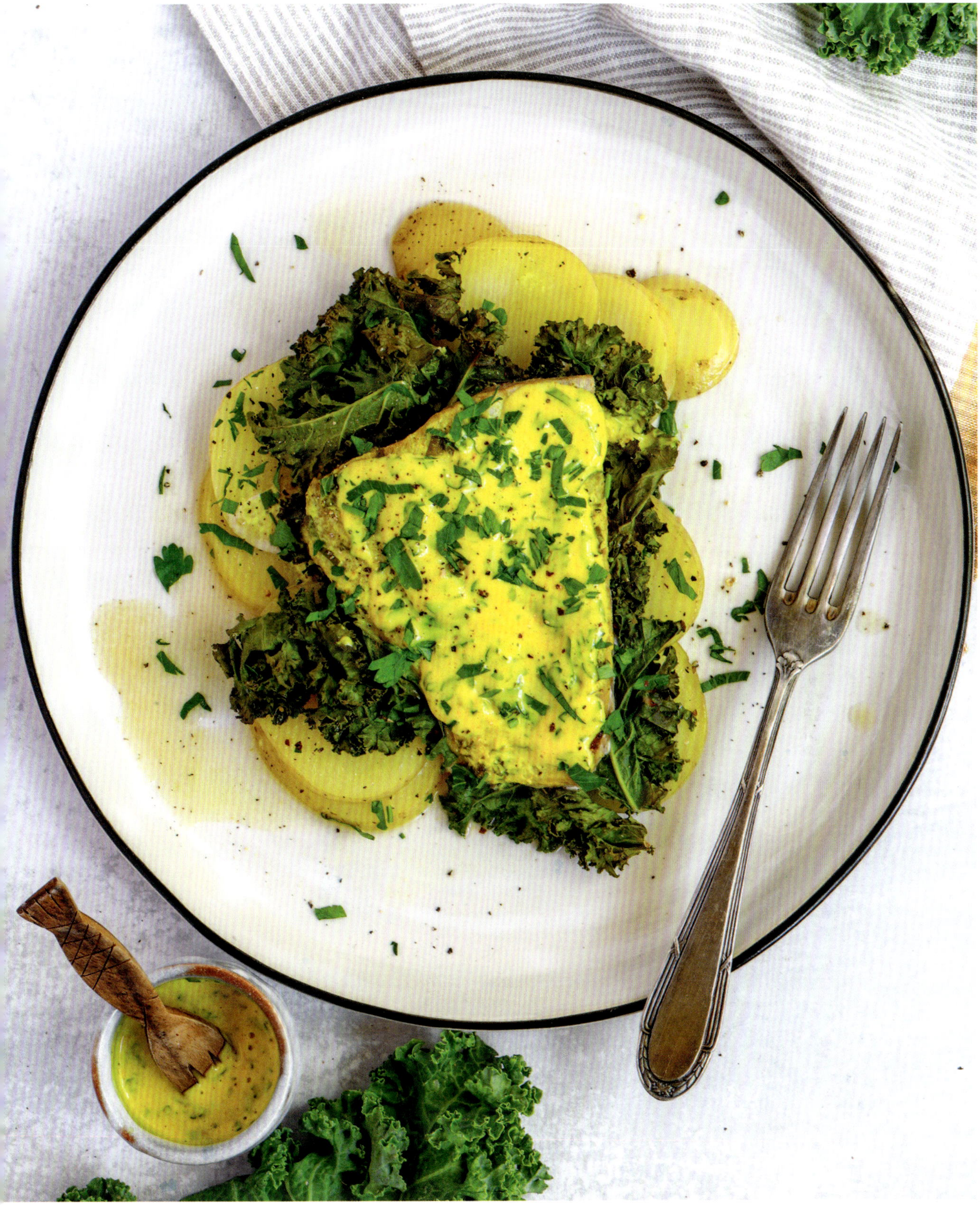

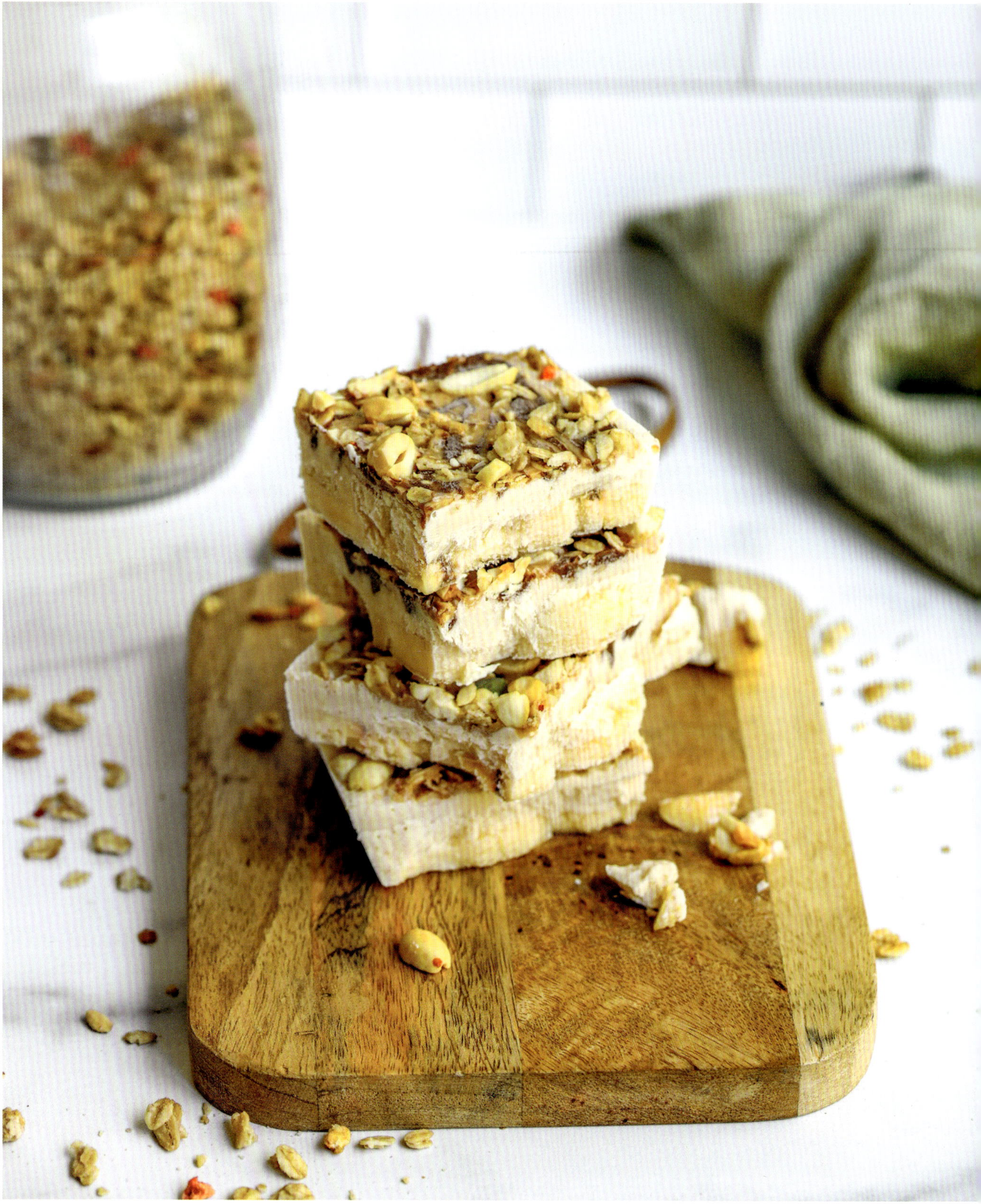

SERVES **8** | **2** HOURS **5** MINUTES

PEANUT BUTTER BANANA COTTAGE CHEESE BARK

INGREDIENTS

2 **bananas**, sliced
1 lb (450 g) **cottage cheese**
3 tbsp **peanut butter**, divided
1 tbsp **honey**
1 tsp **vanilla extract**
2 tbsp **chocolate chips**, melted
3 tbsp **granola**
2 tbsp **peanuts**, chopped flaky sea salt (optional)

METHOD

- Line a rimmed baking sheet with parchment paper or a silicone liner. Arrange the banana slices in a rectangle (approx. 35 slices, 5x7 layout).
- Place the cottage cheese, 2 tablespoons of peanut butter, honey and vanilla extract into a blender, or food processor, and blend until smooth.
- Pour the mixture over the bananas and spread it into an even layer. Drizzle the remaining tablespoon of peanut butter on top.
- Melt the chocolate chips in the microwave, stirring every 30 seconds until smooth (about 60–90 seconds in total). Drizzle the chocolate in a zigzag pattern over the bark.
- Sprinkle over the granola, chopped peanuts, and a small pinch of flaky sea salt (optional).
- Place into the freezer for at least 2 hours, or until fully frozen. Break the bark into pieces by hand or cut into chunks with a knife.

STORAGE

- Store in a freezer-safe container or Ziploc bag for up to 3 months.

ENERGY: **193** kcal	CARBS: **19** g	PROTEIN: **9** g	FAT: **9** g

SERVES **8** | **1** HOUR **10** MINUTES

SALTED CINNAMON PROTEIN BARS

INGREDIENTS

4 oz (40 g) **vanilla whey protein powder**
1 tsp **cinnamon**
3.5 oz (100 g) **rolled oats**
2 tbsp **coconut oil**, melted
4.2 oz (120 g) **natural almond butter**
2.6 oz (75 g) **honey flaky sea salt**

METHOD

- In a food processor fitted with a steel S blade, add the protein powder, cinnamon, and rolled oats. Blend for 1 minute until the oats are powdery and fine.
- Add the melted coconut oil, almond butter, honey, and vanilla extract to the food processor. Blend for another 30 seconds until the mixture is well combined.
- Fold some of the mixture in your hand; it should form a ball and not crumble. If the mixture is crumbly, add 1 tbsp water and process again.
- Line a 9 x 5 inch loaf pan with parchment paper, and press the protein bar mixture into the pan. Sprinkle with flaky sea salt, then chill for 2 hours.
- Remove the bars from the loaf pan and cut them into 8 squares.

ENERGY: **220** kcal | CARBS: **19** g | PROTEIN: **9** g | FAT: **12** g

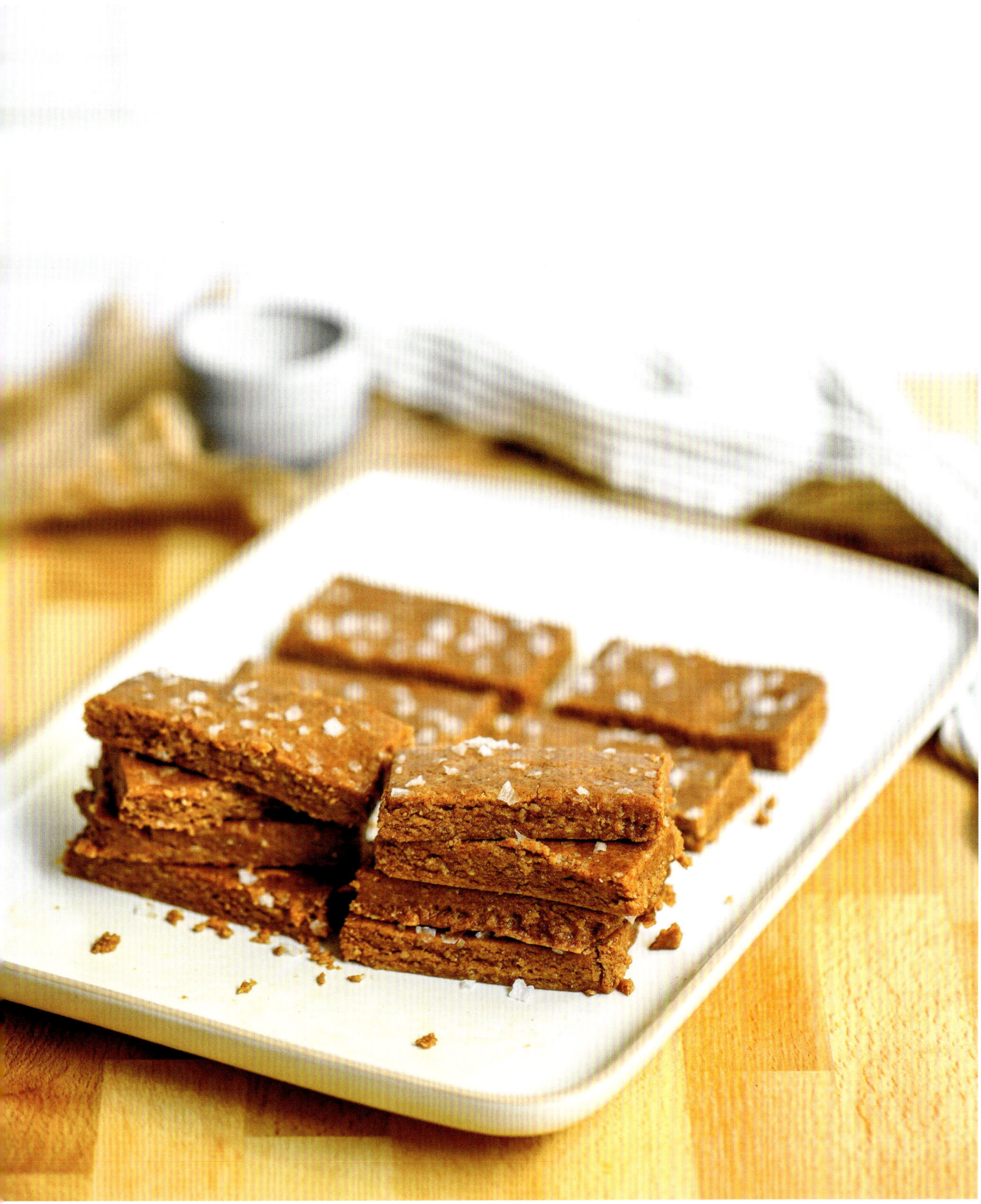

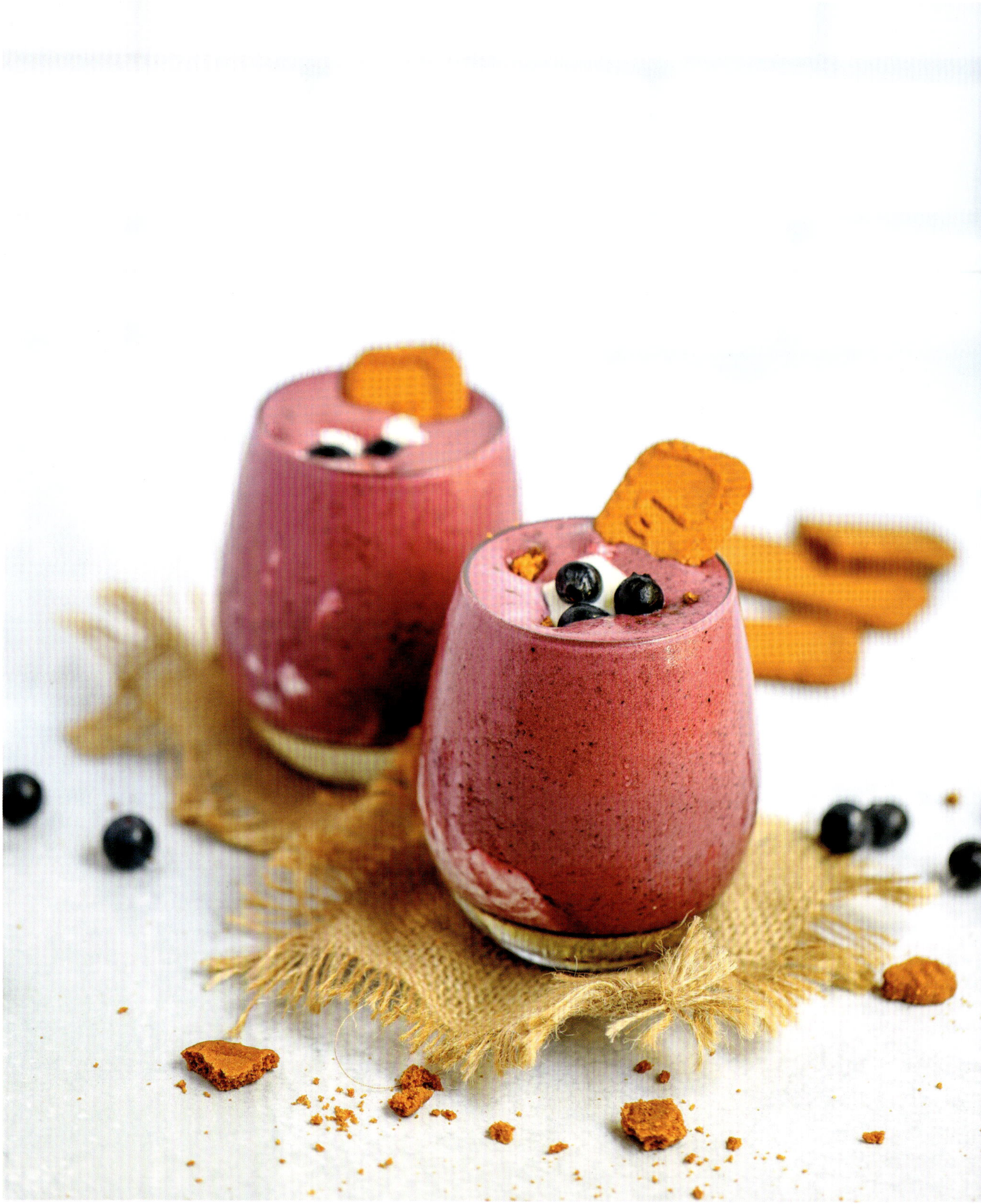

SERVES **2** | **5** MINUTES

BLUEBERRY CHEESECAKE PROTEIN SMOOTHIE

INGREDIENTS

7.9 oz (225 g) **frozen blueberries**
8 oz (240 ml) **unsweetened vanilla almond milk**
4 oz (115 g) **Greek yogurt**
1 oz (30 g) **vanilla protein powder**
2 tbsp **cream cheese**

To serve (optional)

2 tbsp **Greek yogurt**
4 **lotus biscuits**
blueberries

METHOD

- Place all the ingredients into a high-speed blender and blend until smooth. Divide equally between 2 glasses and serve.

OPTIONAL

- Top with more yogurt, blueberries and lotus biscuits before serving (not included in nutritional breakdown).

ENERGY: **227** kcal	CARBS: **21** g	PROTEIN: **20** g	FAT: **7** g

CHAPTER 5

MANAGING COMMON PERIMENOPAUSE CHALLENGES THROUGH DIET AND LIFESTYLE

Perimenopause brings with it a unique set of challenges, but understanding how to manage these through diet and lifestyle can make all the difference in how you feel. From mood swings and anxiety to weight fluctuations and hot flashes, each symptom has a root cause tied to the hormonal changes happening in your body. By making small adjustments to what you eat and how you approach daily routines, you can alleviate many of these common symptoms, allowing you to navigate this stage with greater ease, balance, and confidence.

Mood swings and anxiety

Mood swings and increased anxiety are some of the most widely reported symptoms of perimenopause. These shifts in mood are often the result of fluctuating estrogen and progesterone levels, which affect neurotransmitters like serotonin and dopamine, the chemicals that help regulate mood and feelings of well-being. Although these hormonal changes are natural, there are ways to support your emotional balance and reduce the intensity of mood swings.

- **Omega-3 fatty acids**: Omega-3s, found in fatty fish, like salmon, mackerel, and sardines, as well as in plant sources like flaxseeds, chia seeds, and walnuts, have been shown to reduce symptoms of anxiety and depression by supporting brain health. Starting the day with an omega-3-rich breakfast – such as a smoothie with chia seeds or a slice of avocado toast topped with smoked salmon – can help regulate mood throughout the day.
- **Magnesium and zinc**: Magnesium, often called the "calming mineral," plays a critical role in stress management and relaxation. Foods rich in magnesium, like leafy greens, pumpkin seeds, and almonds, are great for reducing anxiety. Similarly, zinc, found in nuts and seeds, eggs, and legumes, supports the nervous system and can reduce stress. Try including a small magnesium-rich snack like a handful of pumpkin seeds or a bowl of Greek yogurt with almonds to give your mood an extra boost.

- **Leafy greens**: Dark, leafy greens like spinach, kale, and Swiss chard are packed with B vitamins, which are essential for energy production and mental clarity. Including a side of greens with lunch or dinner can help stabilise your mood, especially when combined with omega-3s or other stress-relieving foods.

Simple dietary changes like these can make a noticeable difference in managing mood swings. Consistency is key; by regularly including these mood-supporting foods, you're giving your brain the resources it needs to stay balanced and resilient in the face of hormonal changes.

Weight fluctuations

Many women experience weight gain during perimenopause, particularly around the abdomen. This is often due to a slower metabolism combined with changes in fat distribution caused by hormonal fluctuations. While weight gain can be frustrating, there are ways to support a healthy weight without restrictive dieting, which can actually backfire by increasing cravings and making it harder to maintain a balanced mood.

- **Fibre-rich foods**: Foods high in fibre, such as vegetables, whole grains, legumes, and fruits, are incredibly beneficial for weight management. Fibre helps you feel full for longer, which can prevent overeating, and it also stabilises blood sugar, reducing cravings for sugary snacks. Start each meal with a portion of fibre-rich vegetables – such as a salad with mixed greens and chopped veggies or a bowl of vegetable soup – to naturally reduce the amount of higher-calorie foods you consume.
- **Lean proteins**: Including lean proteins like chicken, fish, tofu, and legumes with each meal can help you stay full and support muscle maintenance, which is essential for a healthy metabolism. Protein stabilises blood sugar, preventing the highs and lows that can lead to cravings and mood swings. Try pairing a portion of lean protein with a high-fibre food for meals that keep you energised and satisfied.
- **Mindful eating practices**: Practising mindfulness when eating can also support weight management. Slow down, savour each bite, and listen to your body's hunger and fullness cues. This practice not only helps with portion control but also makes meals more satisfying, allowing you to enjoy food without the risk of overeating. Set aside distractions while you eat and take a few deep breaths before beginning your meal to focus on the experience.

By incorporating fibre, lean protein, and mindfulness, you can stabilise your weight and improve your relationship with food. These changes will support a healthy metabolism, helping you feel more comfortable and confident in your body as it adjusts to new hormonal patterns.

Hot flashes and night sweats

Hot flashes and night sweats are among the most uncomfortable and disruptive symptoms of perimenopause. Characterised by sudden, intense waves of heat, often accompanied by sweating and flushed skin, hot flashes can occur anytime, day or night. While they're largely due to hormonal fluctuations, certain dietary and lifestyle changes can help reduce their frequency and severity.

- **Cooling foods**: Foods like cucumbers, melons, celery, and leafy greens have natural cooling properties that help regulate body temperature. Including a cucumber or melon salad at lunch or snacking on celery sticks in the afternoon can provide natural relief from heat. These foods also help with hydration, which is essential for reducing hot flashes.
- **Herbal teas**: Some herbal teas, such as peppermint, sage, and chamomile, have natural cooling and calming effects. Sage, in particular, has been shown to reduce the intensity of hot flashes. Enjoying a cup of peppermint or sage tea in the evening can help cool your body and prepare you for a more restful night's sleep. Chamomile tea, with its calming properties, is another great choice, especially if stress or anxiety trigger hot flashes for you.
- **Avoiding triggers**: Certain foods and drinks, like spicy foods, caffeine, and alcohol, can trigger hot flashes by increasing blood flow and body temperature. By identifying and avoiding specific triggers, you can reduce the likelihood of experiencing hot flashes. Try keeping a symptom journal, noting when you have a hot flash and what you ate or drank beforehand. This can help you identify patterns and make informed dietary choices.

Making small adjustments to your diet and daily routine can provide significant relief from hot flashes and night sweats. By incorporating cooling foods and herbal teas and avoiding known triggers, you're actively taking steps to regain control over your comfort.

Energy and fatigue

Fatigue is another common complaint during perimenopause, often resulting from poor sleep quality, hormonal changes, and a slowed metabolism. However, certain foods and lifestyle practices can provide a natural energy boost, helping you feel more refreshed and ready to face the day.

- **Iron-rich foods**: Iron deficiency can lead to feelings of fatigue and lethargy, so it's important to include iron-rich foods like lean meats, lentils, spinach, and pumpkin seeds in your diet. Pairing these with vitamin C-rich foods, like bell peppers or citrus fruits, can help enhance iron absorption. Starting the day with a spinach and bell pepper omelette, for example, is a great way to combine these nutrients for a morning energy boost.

- **B Vitamins**: B vitamins play a key role in energy production. Foods high in B vitamins – like whole grains, eggs, and leafy greens – support sustained energy throughout the day. Including a variety of B-vitamin-rich foods in your meals can combat fatigue and keep you mentally sharp.
- **Hydration**: Dehydration can cause fatigue, so make sure you're drinking plenty of water throughout the day. Herbal teas and water-rich foods like cucumbers and melons also contribute to hydration. Keeping a water bottle with you can help remind you to drink regularly, which is particularly important if you're prone to hot flashes that lead to fluid loss.

By incorporating iron, B vitamins, and staying well-hydrated, you're actively supporting your body's energy levels. These small changes can help you combat fatigue, improving your ability to stay focused and active.

Bloating and digestion

Digestive issues, like bloating and irregularity, are common during perimenopause. Hormonal changes can affect gut motility and microbiome balance, leading to discomfort and bloating. However, by focusing on anti-inflammatory and probiotic-rich foods, you can support your gut health and reduce these symptoms.

- **Probiotic-rich foods**: Probiotics found in yogurt, kefir, sauerkraut, and kimchi support a healthy gut microbiome, which is essential for digestion and reducing bloating. Including a serving of probiotic-rich foods each day can improve gut health and relieve digestive discomfort. Try adding a small bowl of Greek yogurt with a sprinkle of berries or incorporating a side of sauerkraut with your lunch.
- **Anti-inflammatory foods**: Foods with anti-inflammatory properties, like turmeric, ginger, and leafy greens, can soothe the digestive tract and reduce bloating. Adding turmeric to soups or stews, or drinking ginger tea after meals, can ease digestion and promote gut comfort.
- **High-fibre foods**: Fibre is crucial for regularity, and foods like whole grains, vegetables, and fruits help promote a healthy digestive system. Aim to include a mix of soluble fibre (found in oats, apples, and beans) and insoluble fibre (found in whole grains and vegetables) to keep things moving smoothly.

By focusing on gut-friendly foods, you can support digestion, reduce bloating, and improve overall comfort. A healthy gut not only alleviates physical discomfort but also contributes to better mental clarity and emotional stability, making it easier to manage your day.

CHAPTER 6

LIFESTYLE TIPS TO SUPPORT A SMOOTH PERIMENOPAUSE TRANSITION

Embracing lifestyle changes during perimenopause can provide a foundation of strength, resilience, and balance that benefits both body and mind. With a focus on movement, mindfulness, sleep, and self-awareness, this chapter offers practical lifestyle strategies to support a smooth transition through perimenopause. By prioritising these aspects of health, you're setting yourself up to navigate this phase with greater comfort, clarity, and confidence.

Exercise for strength and balance

Regular exercise is one of the most effective ways to support your body during perimenopause. Movement not only strengthens muscles and supports bone density but also enhances mood, reduces stress, and sharpens mental clarity. Including a variety of exercises that focus on strength, flexibility, and balance can help you stay physically resilient and mentally engaged.

- **Strength training**: As estrogen levels decline, bone density and muscle mass can decrease, making it important to focus on exercises that help maintain strength. Strength training, such as weightlifting or bodyweight exercises (like squats and lunges), supports bone density, reduces the risk of osteoporosis, and boosts metabolism. Start with light weights or resistance bands, and gradually increase the intensity as you feel more comfortable. Just two or three sessions per week can make a big difference in muscle tone and bone health.
- **Yoga**: Yoga combines physical movement with mindfulness, helping to improve flexibility, balance, and stress resilience. The gentle stretching in yoga also reduces muscle tension, which can be particularly beneficial if you experience stiffness or joint pain. Yoga poses like Warrior II, Tree Pose, and Downward Dog are effective for building both strength and balance. Try to incorporate yoga a few times a week, even if it's just a short session, to reap the mental and physical benefits.

- **Walking**: Walking is a low-impact, accessible exercise that promotes cardiovascular health, aids in weight management, and boosts mood. A 30-minute walk each day can enhance endurance, mental clarity, and mood by increasing the release of endorphins, the body's natural mood-boosting chemicals. Walking outdoors in nature also provides the added benefit of fresh air and can be a wonderful way to reduce stress. Aim to walk at a moderate pace to elevate your heart rate without straining.

By integrating these forms of exercise into your weekly routine, you're supporting your body's resilience and creating a foundation of strength and balance that will carry you through perimenopause and beyond. Consistency is key; even moderate amounts of movement can have a profound effect on your overall health and well-being.

Mindfulness and stress relief

Perimenopause often brings emotional shifts that can feel overwhelming. Incorporating mindfulness practices is a powerful way to manage stress, enhance emotional stability, and improve resilience. Simple, daily mindfulness practices allow you to stay present and grounded, reducing the impact of stress on both your body and mind.

- **Breathing exercises**: Conscious breathing helps calm the nervous system, promoting relaxation and reducing anxiety. One effective technique is called "4-7-8 breathing," where you inhale for four counts, hold for seven, and exhale for eight. Practising this for just a few minutes can help alleviate tension and bring you into a more relaxed state. Try incorporating this breathing exercise whenever you feel anxious or before bedtime to aid in sleep.
- **Meditation**: Meditation doesn't require any special equipment or setup, just a few quiet minutes each day. Start with a simple, five-minute meditation where you focus on your breath, letting thoughts come and go without judgment. Meditation trains the mind to stay present, which can reduce reactivity to stressors and improve emotional balance. Apps like *Headspace* or *Calm* offer guided meditations if you're new to the practice and looking for direction.
- **Mindful movement**: Bringing mindfulness into daily movement – whether through yoga, walking, or even simple stretches – allows you to focus on your body's sensations, letting go of distractions and stress. This practice encourages you to tune into your body and its needs, building a stronger mind-body connection that promotes mental clarity and relaxation.

These mindfulness practices are small but mighty tools for reducing stress and enhancing emotional stability. By prioritising these practices, you're equipping yourself with techniques to manage perimenopausal challenges with greater ease and peace.

Sleep optimisation

Sleep can become elusive during perimenopause due to hormonal shifts that disrupt the body's natural rhythms. Poor sleep quality can lead to intensified fatigue, mood swings, and stress. Creating a supportive sleep routine is essential, and timing meals can also play a significant role in promoting restful sleep. Here, we'll explore dietary and lifestyle tips, including the importance of intermittent fasting and meal timing, to help you optimise your sleep quality.

- **Intermittent fasting and sleep**: Intermittent fasting (IF), which involves restricting eating to certain hours of the day and fasting during the remaining hours, can be highly beneficial for improving sleep and overall health. By eating within a specific window, such as an 8-hour period during the day, the body is given a longer fasting period, which allows for better digestion and metabolic regulation. This fasting period may support more restful sleep by reducing late-night digestive activity and helping the body maintain stable blood sugar levels overnight.
  IF has also been shown to promote the release of human growth hormone and enhance cellular repair processes, both of which are active during sleep. For perimenopausal women, intermittent fasting may help stabilise insulin levels, reduce inflammation, and manage weight, which collectively contribute to better sleep and overall balance. Starting with a 12-hour eating window (e.g., 8 am to 8 pm) and gradually shortening it as you feel comfortable can help you ease into IF without feeling deprived.

- **Benefits of not eating too late**: Eating late in the evening can interfere with sleep quality by activating the digestive system when it should be winding down. Large, heavy meals close to bedtime can cause discomfort, indigestion, and even acid reflux, which makes it harder to fall asleep and stay asleep. Additionally, late-night eating can disrupt the body's natural circadian rhythms, leading to heightened alertness just when you're trying to relax.
  Having your last meal at least 3–4 hours before bedtime gives your body adequate time to digest and allows your metabolism to naturally slow down for the night. By avoiding late-night eating, you reduce the likelihood of blood sugar spikes and crashes, which can trigger midnight wake-ups and restless sleep. Finishing dinner earlier also allows for the natural release of melatonin, the hormone that signals it's time for sleep, promoting a smoother transition into restful sleep.

- **Pre-bedtime snacks (if needed)**: While intermittent fasting discourages late-night eating, if you find that hunger disrupts your sleep, a light, sleep-supportive snack 3–4 hours before bed can be helpful. Choose snacks rich in magnesium, such as a small handful of almonds or a banana, to ease muscle tension and calm the nervous system. Alternatively, a cup of chamomile tea or a glass of warm milk with a sprinkle of cinnamon can create a relaxing pre-sleep ritual without adding digestive strain.

- **Reducing stimulants**: Stimulants like caffeine and alcohol can interfere with sleep quality, so limit these in the hours leading up to bedtime. Avoid caffeine after 1pm to prevent restless sleep and consider replacing an evening glass of wine with herbal tea to help your body relax naturally.

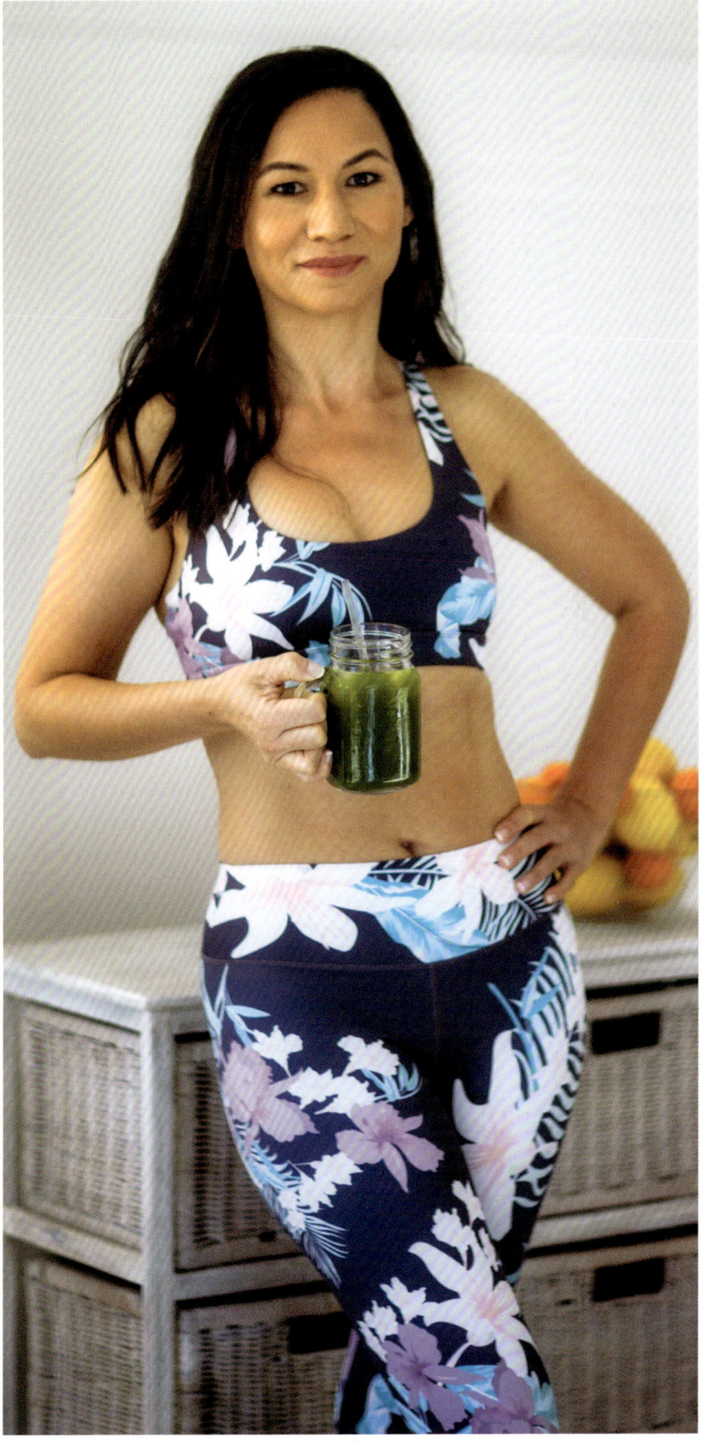

By incorporating intermittent fasting, avoiding late meals, and choosing light, calming snacks if needed, you're setting yourself up for more restful sleep. These habits support the body's natural rhythms, reduce sleep disruptions, and create a balanced approach to evening nourishment. Prioritising sleep optimisation helps you wake up feeling refreshed and ready to face the day, empowering you to handle perimenopausal challenges with energy and clarity.

Tracking and adapting

Perimenopause is a dynamic process, with symptoms that can fluctuate from week to week. Tracking your symptoms, diet, and lifestyle habits is an effective way to identify patterns, make adjustments, and better understand how your body responds to different approaches. This self-awareness not only helps you adapt your habits to better manage symptoms but also empowers you to feel more in control of your health.

- **Symptom journal**: Keeping a journal of your daily symptoms allows you to monitor changes over time and track improvements. Note things like mood, energy levels, sleep quality, hot flashes, and any other physical or emotional symptoms you experience. By looking back over your journal, you may notice patterns that can inform your dietary or lifestyle adjustments.
- **Diet and activity log**: In addition to tracking symptoms, keeping a record of what you eat, when you exercise, and how you sleep can provide valuable insights. For example, you may find that including certain foods, like leafy greens or omega-3s, positively impacts your mood, or that exercising earlier in the day improves sleep. This data helps you make informed decisions about what changes are working for you and which may need further adjustment.
- **Adjusting habits**: As you track your progress, be open to adapting your routines based on what you observe. If certain foods consistently trigger symptoms like bloating or mood swings, try adjusting your diet accordingly. Similarly, if a particular exercise or mindfulness practice leaves you feeling especially calm or energised, consider making it a more regular part of your routine. Tracking and adapting allows you to make perimenopause a personalised journey of discovery.

By staying in tune with your body and observing how different factors influence your symptoms, you're actively participating in your own well-being. This awareness not only helps you manage current symptoms but also equips you with tools to maintain a balanced, healthy lifestyle beyond perimenopause.

Moving into menopause and beyond doesn't have to be a daunting experience. By maintaining the healthy habits developed during perimenopause, staying active, eating nourishing foods, and nurturing your emotional health, you can approach this phase with strength, balance, and optimism. Establishing a support network of family, friends, and community connections further enhances your journey, providing encouragement and shared experiences that make the transition smoother. Embracing these tools and strategies not only supports you now but also sets the foundation for a vibrant, fulfilling life well into the years ahead.

EMBRACING MENOPAUSE WITH CONFIDENCE AND VITALITY

As I sat down to write *The Perimenopause Plan*, I reflected deeply on my own journey through perimenopause and the ways I've managed this profound transition. Like many of you, I faced the surprise of unexpected changes – mood swings, night sweats, shifts in energy, and a body that felt foreign at times. It was in those moments that I turned to the practices I share in this book. Each tip, each meal plan, each mindfulness exercise has been my own lifeline, helping me feel more grounded, balanced, and hopeful.

Moving into menopause and beyond doesn't have to be daunting. While it is a significant life transition, it's also an opportunity to embrace a new chapter with vitality, resilience, and a sense of purpose. I'm living proof that by maintaining the healthy habits developed during perimenopause, nurturing your emotional health, and fostering connections with those around you, this stage of life can feel empowering.

Maintaining healthy habits

The routines we create in perimenopause are gifts we give to our future selves. As I've navigated this journey, staying active, eating nourishing foods, and dedicating time to self-care have made all the difference. Regular movement, whether through gentle yoga, brisk walks, or strength training, has helped me stay physically strong and mentally clear. I can't emphasise enough how much energy and positivity come from just a little movement each day. These habits have been a touchstone in my life, reminding me that I'm supporting my body in the best way I know how.

Balanced nutrition is another foundation that has kept me feeling energised and stable. Embracing whole foods, colourful vegetables, lean proteins, and healthy fats has become a way to nurture myself daily. Each meal becomes an act of self-care, and I know that by choosing foods rich in calcium, magnesium, omega-3s, and fibre, I'm building a foundation for long-term health. I've found that these nourishing foods have given me more than just physical strength – they've lifted my mood, kept my energy stable, and helped me feel grounded.

And let's not forget the power of mindfulness and stress relief. Taking a few moments each day to focus on my breath, practice gratitude, or simply pause has become essential. Mindfulness has allowed me to experience perimenopause as a phase of growth and understanding. I hope that you, too, will find that these practices help you feel more resilient and prepared for each day. These aren't just habits – they are small, sacred acts of self-care that bring comfort and stability, especially in moments of change.

Embracing the transition with positivity

Transitioning into menopause is something I've come to view with a sense of acceptance and even excitement. I know that for many of us, there's a bit of fear about this transition, wondering what's next or how life might look on the other side. But let me share what I've learned: each phase of life brings with it a unique beauty and strength. Menopause marks a new beginning, one where we are free from the cycles of our younger years and can embrace a lifestyle focused on well-being and self-discovery.

One of the most surprising gifts of this journey has been a sense of clarity and purpose. Moving through perimenopause and into menopause has encouraged me to truly focus on what matters most in life. This clarity has allowed me to let go of habits, routines, or beliefs that no longer serve me, and to welcome new practices that support my health, happiness, and growth. I encourage you to approach this transition with an open heart, knowing that it's an opportunity to create the lifestyle you want.

Creating a support network

Navigating perimenopause and menopause can feel isolating at times, but I've found incredible strength in leaning on those around me. Establishing a support network of family, friends, and like-minded women has been one of the most comforting and empowering parts of this experience. Sharing stories, laughter, advice, and even the occasional tear has made the journey feel so much lighter and has reminded me that I'm not alone.

My close friends, who are also experiencing this transition, have been a source of wisdom and encouragement. We openly discuss our experiences, share tips, and, most importantly, remind each other to laugh through the ups and downs. Finding this connection has been invaluable. Whether it's a weekly walk with a friend, a family gathering, or an online community, reaching out and sharing your journey with others can make all the difference.

If you're feeling uncertain about this transition, I encourage you to find those connections, even if it's just one person to share with. There are so many wonderful communities out there – both online and offline – where you'll find empathy, advice, and the companionship of others on the same path. Building these connections isn't just about managing symptoms; it's about celebrating this life phase together and embracing all it has to offer.

Finding "me time" and the value of escape

As women, we often find ourselves caring for everyone else – our families, our work commitments, our friendships – sometimes at the expense of our own needs. During perimenopause and menopause, carving out "me time" becomes more than just a luxury; it's a necessity for mental clarity, emotional balance, and physical well-being. I know firsthand how challenging it can be to find that space, but I've come to realise just how transformative it is.

One of the best ways I've found to truly reset and reconnect with myself is by taking a retreat. Stepping away from the daily routine, even just for a weekend, can offer a chance to unwind, reflect, and focus solely on my well-being. Whether it's a yoga retreat, a quiet nature getaway, or a wellness retreat focused on self-care, these experiences allow me to recharge in ways that daily "me time" at home simply can't provide.

A retreat, even a short one, can also give you a new perspective on your routines and help you set fresh goals for health, relaxation, and personal growth. It's a chance to be surrounded by like-minded women, all focusing on self-care, and it provides a peaceful environment to reflect without the distractions of daily life.

If you're able to, consider planning a retreat away from family responsibilities, just to focus on *you*. It's a gift to yourself that benefits not only your well-being but also your relationships, as you return feeling renewed and ready to face life with a fresh sense of energy and calm. Remember, your "me time" isn't selfish – it's an essential part of thriving during this transition. Embrace it as a beautiful part of your journey, and let it be something you prioritise with joy and intention.

Looking to the future with confidence

As I move forward in my journey, I am filled with gratitude for the lessons that perimenopause has taught me and the strength I've gained. I've come to see this phase as a powerful reminder of how resilient we are and how capable we are of adapting to change. My hope is that you, too, will feel empowered as you step into menopause and beyond, knowing that you have the tools, knowledge, and support to thrive.

Each chapter in this book has been crafted with care, rooted in my own experiences and the experiences of countless women who have walked this path. I hope these insights, tips, and routines help you approach perimenopause and menopause with a sense of control and clarity. Remember that your health, happiness, and well-being are in your hands, and each small act of self-care adds up to create a vibrant, fulfilling life.

Menopause isn't an end – it's the beginning of a new chapter filled with freedom, wisdom, and joy. By sustaining the habits you've nurtured, by prioritising your health and well-being, and by leaning on those around you, this transition can be one of the most rewarding and enriching times of your life. I am honoured to have been part of your journey, and I look forward to the vibrant, balanced life that lies ahead for you. Here's to embracing this next chapter with confidence, grace, and endless possibility.

RECIPE INDEX

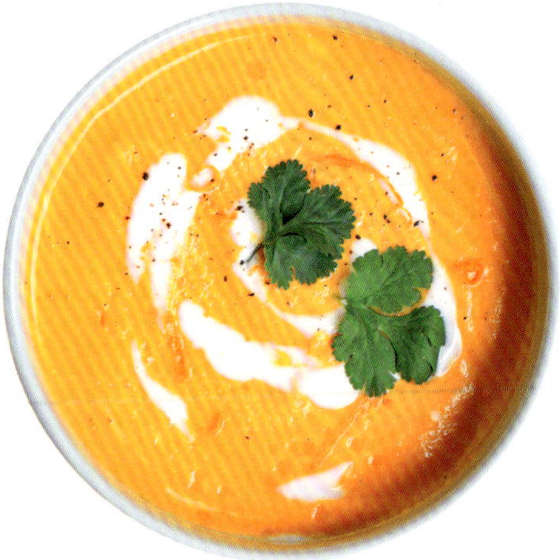

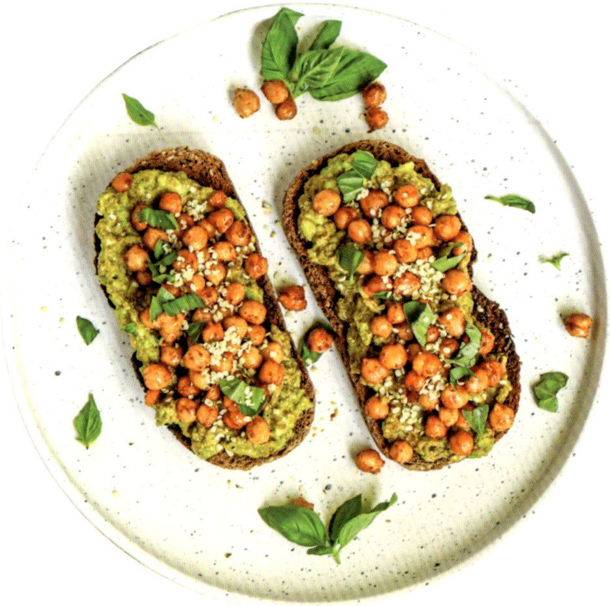

First published in 2025 by New Holland Publishers
Sydney

newhollandpublishers.com

A record of this book is held at the National Library of Australia.

ISBN 9781760797904

Text: Faye James
Photography: Exceed and Darrin James
Recipe development: Faye James
Managing Director: Fiona Schultz
Designer: Andrew Davies
Production Director: Arlene Gippert

Printed in China

Keep up with New Holland Publishers:
NewHollandPublishers
@newhollandpublishers

US $19.99
UK £14.99

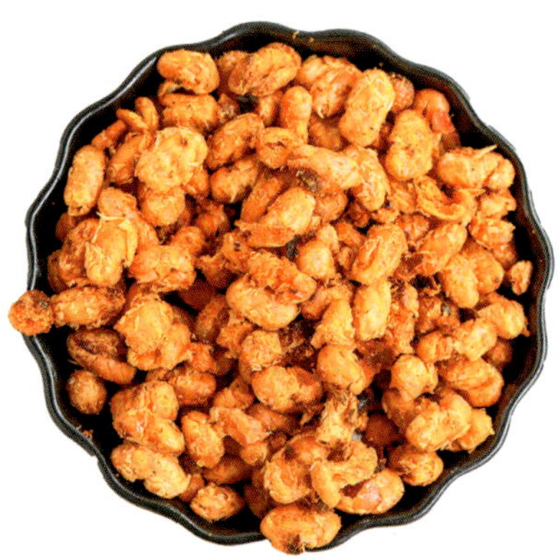